CROHN'S DISEASE

COOKBOOK

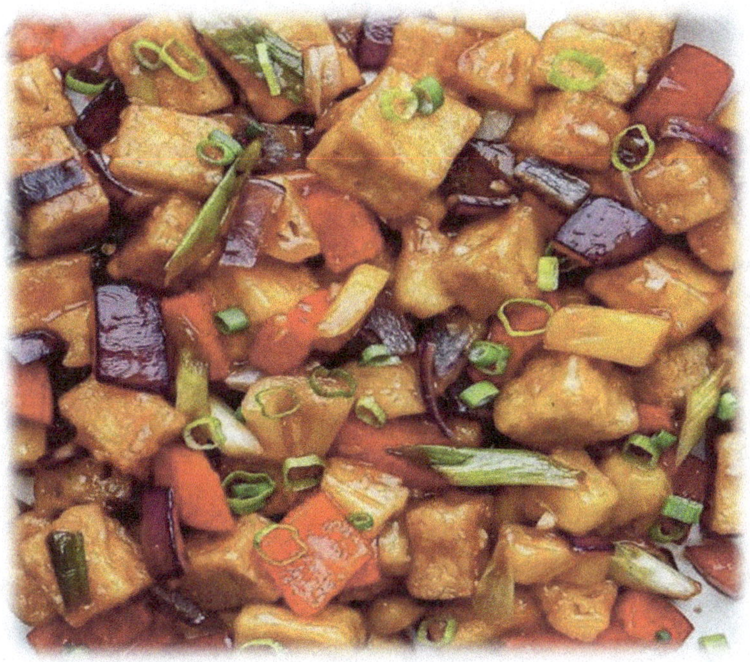

Easy and delicious recipes to relieve inflammatory bowel disease and support digestive wellness

LAKEISHA OWENS

TABLE OF CONTENT

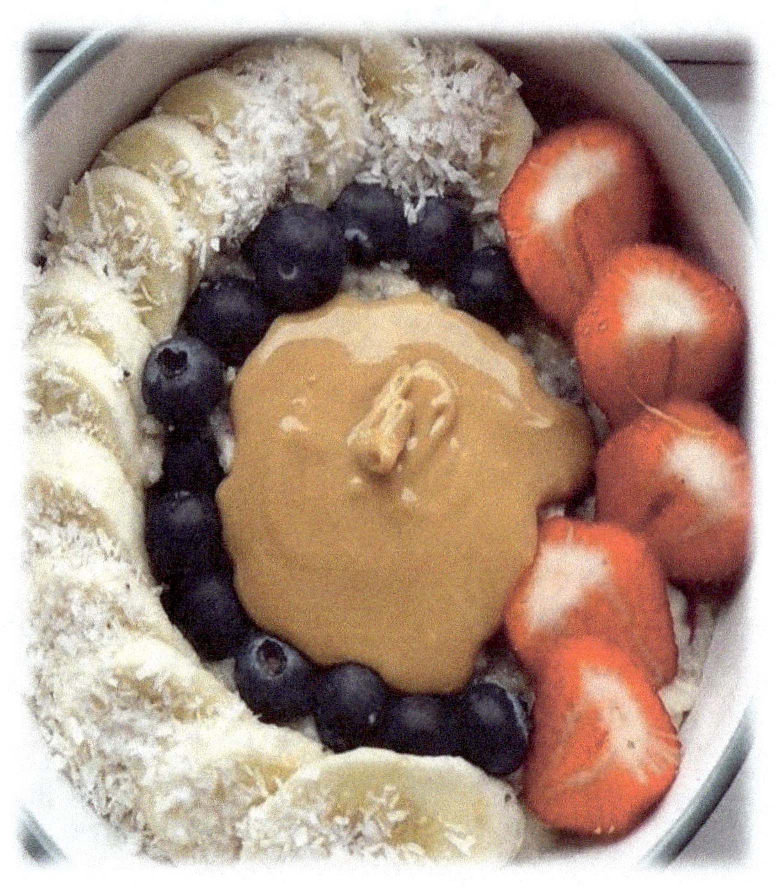

INTRODUCTION

An inflammatory bowel disorder that affects millions worldwide, Crohn's demands not only medical attention but also a holistic approach to nourishment. Recognizing the pivotal role that diet plays in mitigating symptoms and enhancing overall well-being, we present **"Crohn's Disease Cookbook."**

This book is not just a collection of recipes; it is a guide crafted with empathy and expertise, aiming to empower individuals living with Crohn's to take control of their culinary journey. Our journey begins with an exploration of the unique relationship between nutrition and Crohn's disease. Delving into the latest scientific research and expert insights, we unravel the mysteries of how specific foods can either trigger or alleviate symptoms. From this foundation, we embark on a culinary adventure, carefully curating a collection of recipes that prioritize not only taste but also the nutritional needs of those with Crohn's.

Each recipe is meticulously crafted, considering the dietary restrictions commonly associated with Crohn's, such as the avoidance of certain fibers, lactose, and trigger foods. Our goal is to offer a diverse array of flavorful dishes that cater to a spectrum of tastes and preferences while keeping in mind the nutritional requirements essential for managing Crohn's symptoms.

Beyond the kitchen, **"Crohn's Disease Cookbook"** equips readers with practical tips on meal planning, grocery shopping, and optimizing nutrient absorption. We understand the challenges of maintaining a balanced and enjoyable diet while coping with the unpredictable nature of Crohn's, and we strive to provide a roadmap for success.

Whether you are a newly diagnosed individual seeking guidance or a long-time warrior in the battle against Crohn's, this cookbook is a companion designed to inspire and empower. By embracing a culinary philosophy centered on nourishment and mindful eating, we hope to empower you to not only manage your condition but to thrive in your journey toward wellness.

Welcome to **"Crohn's Disease Cookbook."** May these pages become a source of comfort, inspiration, and, most importantly, a celebration of the remarkable resilience of the human spirit.

CHAPTER 1

UNDERSTANDING CROHN'S DISEASE

Crohn's disease is a chronic inflammatory bowel disorder that significantly impacts the digestive system. Characterized by inflammation of the gastrointestinal tract, Crohn's can affect any part of the digestive system, from the mouth to the anus. Common symptoms include abdominal pain, diarrhea, weight loss, fatigue, and nutritional deficiencies.

The exact cause of Crohn's remains unclear, but it is believed to result from a combination of genetic, environmental, and immune system factors. The immune system mistakenly attacks the healthy cells of the digestive tract, leading to chronic inflammation.

Living with Crohn's often entails navigating dietary challenges, as certain foods can exacerbate symptoms. While there is no one-size-fits-all diet for individuals with Crohn's, common triggers include high-fiber foods, dairy products, spicy foods, and certain fats. A cookbook tailored to Crohn's sufferers should, therefore, provide delicious and nutritious recipes that accommodate these dietary restrictions while promoting overall well-being.

In addition to dietary considerations, managing Crohn's involves medical treatments such as medications, lifestyle adjustments, and, in severe cases, surgery. The unpredictable nature of the disease requires individuals to adopt a proactive and adaptable approach to their health, emphasizing the importance of a supportive and informed community.

The **"Crohn's Disease Cookbook"** aims to be a valuable resource for individuals navigating the culinary aspects of life with Crohn's. By offering a collection of carefully curated recipes and practical tips, this cookbook seeks to empower individuals to make informed and enjoyable food choices that contribute to their overall health and well-being. It is not just a cookbook but a guide that recognizes the nuanced relationship between nutrition and the management of Crohn's disease, aiming to enhance the quality of life for those on their journey to wellness.

WHAT TO EAT AND AVOID

Diet plays a crucial role in managing Crohn's disease, and understanding which foods to include and which to avoid is essential for minimizing symptoms and promoting overall well-being. While individual responses to specific foods may vary, here's a general guide to help those with Crohn's make informed dietary choices:

Foods to Eat:

Low-Fiber Fruits and Vegetables: Opt for well-cooked and peeled fruits and vegetables to reduce fiber content. Examples include bananas, melons, applesauce, carrots, and zucchini.

Lean Proteins: Choose lean sources of protein to support muscle health without aggravating digestive symptoms. Options include skinless poultry, fish, eggs, and tofu.

Low-Fat Dairy or Alternatives: Lactose intolerance is common in individuals with Crohn's, so consider lactose-free dairy or non-dairy alternatives like almond, soy, or lactose-free milk.

Grains and Starches: Stick to refined grains and easily digestible starches such as white rice, white bread, and pasta. These provide energy without causing excess strain on the digestive system.

Nut Butters and Seeds: Smooth nut butters and seedless varieties can be good sources of healthy fats and protein without the irritation caused by whole nuts and seeds.

Well-Cooked Meats: Opt for tender, well-cooked meats to make digestion easier. Ground or minced meats are often better tolerated.

Probiotic-Rich Foods: Incorporate probiotics to promote a healthy gut microbiome. Yogurt with live cultures, kefir, and fermented foods like sauerkraut may be beneficial.

Foods to Avoid:

High-Fiber Foods: Limit or avoid high-fiber foods, including raw fruits and vegetables, whole grains, and legumes, as they can be challenging to digest and may worsen symptoms.

Spicy Foods: Spices and seasonings like pepper, chili, and hot sauces can be irritating to the digestive tract and should be used sparingly.

Dairy Products (if intolerant): If lactose intolerant, minimize or eliminate dairy products. Choose lactose-free options or alternatives like almond or coconut milk.

High-Fat Foods: Greasy or fried foods can contribute to diarrhea and should be consumed in moderation.

Raw Nuts and Seeds: The coarse texture of nuts and seeds may exacerbate digestive issues. Opt for nut butters without added seeds.

Caffeine and Alcohol: Both can be dehydrating and may contribute to gastrointestinal irritation. It's wise to moderate or eliminate these from the diet.

High-Sugar Foods: Excessive sugar can contribute to inflammation and discomfort. Choose low-sugar alternatives and be mindful of processed sweets.

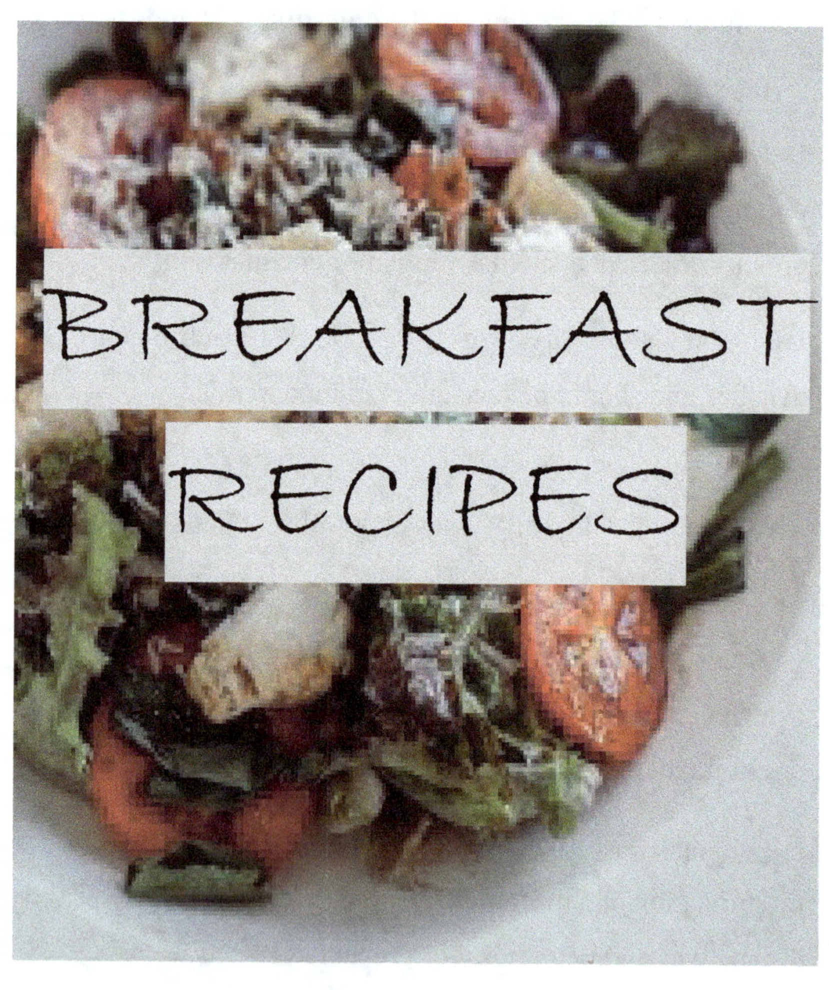

BREAKFAST
RECIPES

CHAPTER 2

BREAKFAST RECIPE

Scrambled Eggs with Spinach and Feta

Ingredients (for 2 servings):

4 eggs

1 cup fresh spinach, chopped

1/4 cup crumbled feta cheese

Salt and pepper to taste

1 tablespoon olive oil

Instructions:

In a bowl, whisk eggs and season with salt and pepper.

Heat olive oil in a pan over medium heat.

Add spinach to the pan and sauté until wilted.

Pour the whisked eggs into the pan and scramble until cooked.

Sprinkle feta cheese over the eggs and stir until melted.

Serve warm.

Nutritional Benefits:

Eggs provide high-quality protein, while spinach offers vitamins and minerals. Feta adds a burst of flavor without being too harsh on the digestive system.

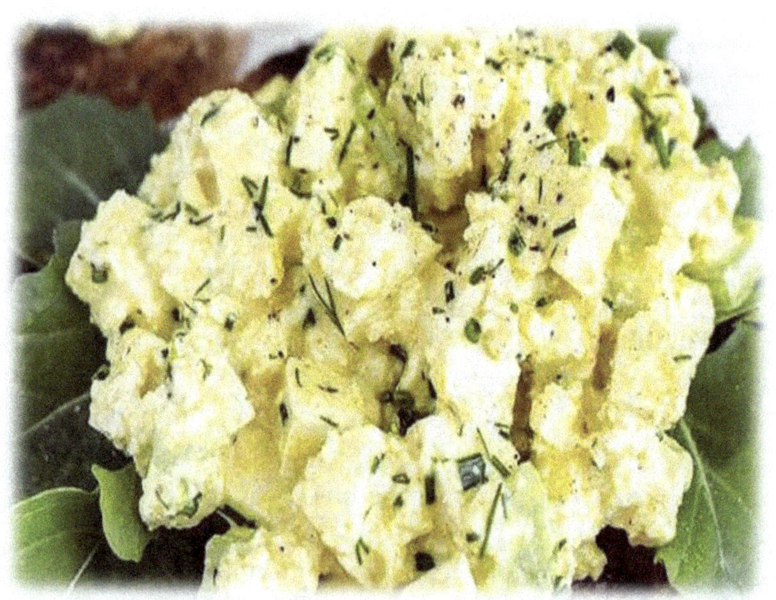

Banana Oatmeal Smoothie Bowl

Ingredients (for 2 servings):

1 cup rolled oats

2 ripe bananas

1 cup almond milk (or lactose-free milk)

2 tablespoons almond butter

1 tablespoon chia seeds

1 teaspoon honey (optional)

Sliced strawberries for topping

Instructions:

In a blender, combine oats, bananas, almond milk, almond butter, chia seeds, and honey.

Blend until smooth and creamy.

Pour the mixture into bowls and top with sliced strawberries.

Serve immediately.

This smoothie bowl provides a good balance of fiber, healthy fats, and protein. Oats and chia seeds are gentle on the digestive system, while bananas offer potassium and natural sweetness.

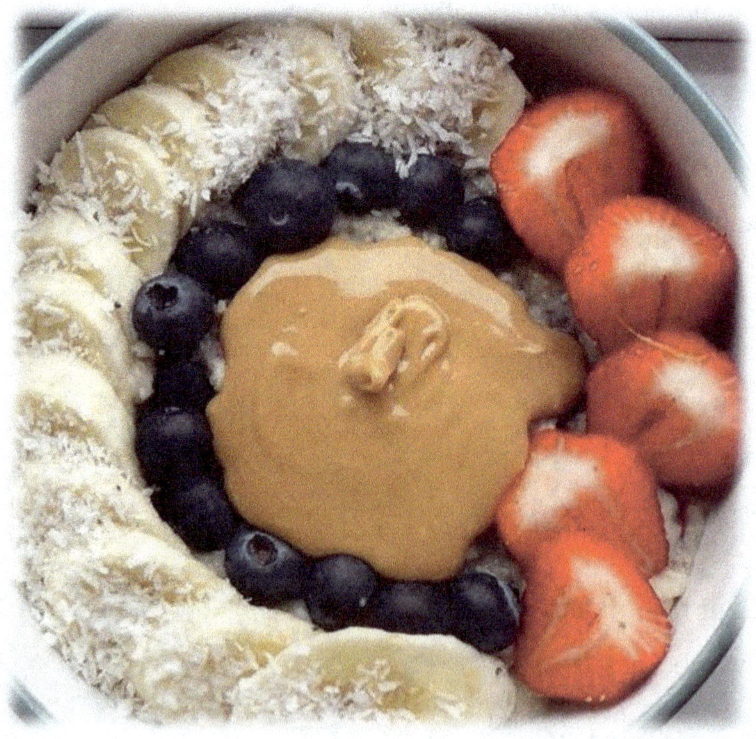

Pumpkin Spice Chia Pudding

Ingredients (for 2 servings):

1/2 cup chia seeds

2 cups almond milk (or lactose-free milk)

1/2 cup canned pumpkin puree

1 teaspoon pumpkin spice

1 tablespoon maple syrup

Chopped walnuts for topping

Instructions:

In a bowl, mix chia seeds, almond milk, pumpkin puree, pumpkin spice, and maple syrup.

Stir well and refrigerate for at least 4 hours or overnight.

Divide into two servings and top with chopped walnuts before serving.

Nutritional Benefits:

Chia seeds provide omega-3 fatty acids and soluble fiber. Pumpkin adds a subtle sweetness and is rich in vitamins A and C.

Greek Yogurt Parfait with Berries

Ingredients (for 2 servings):

1 cup Greek yogurt (lactose-free if needed)

1 cup mixed berries (blueberries, raspberries, strawberries)

1/4 cup granola

1 tablespoon honey (optional)

Instructions:

In two glasses or bowls, layer Greek yogurt, mixed berries, and granola.

Repeat the layers.

Drizzle honey on top if desired.

Serve chilled.

Nutritional Benefits:

Greek yogurt offers probiotics and protein, while berries provide antioxidants. Granola adds crunch and additional fiber.

Quinoa Breakfast Bowl

Ingredients (for 2 servings):

1 cup cooked quinoa

1/2 cup sliced almonds

1/2 cup diced mango

2 tablespoons shredded coconut

1 tablespoon maple syrup

Instructions:

In a bowl, combine cooked quinoa, sliced almonds, diced mango, and shredded coconut.

Drizzle with maple syrup and toss gently.

Divide into two bowls and serve.

Nutritional Benefits:

Quinoa is a good source of protein and fiber. Almonds add healthy fats, while mango provides natural sweetness and vitamins.

Cinnamon Apple Rice Pudding

Ingredients (for 2 servings):

1 cup cooked white rice

1 cup almond milk (or lactose-free milk)

1 apple, peeled and diced

1/2 teaspoon cinnamon

1 tablespoon honey

Chopped pecans for topping

Instructions:

In a saucepan, combine cooked rice, almond milk, diced apple, cinnamon, and honey.

Simmer over low heat, stirring occasionally, until the mixture thickens.

Divide into two bowls and top with chopped pecans before serving.

Nutritional Benefits:

Rice provides easily digestible carbohydrates, while apples offer fiber and a hint of natural sweetness. Cinnamon adds flavor without added sugar.

Salmon and Avocado Breakfast Wrap

Ingredients (for 2 servings):

2 whole-grain tortillas

1/2-pound smoked salmon

1 avocado, sliced

1/4 cup cream cheese (lactose-free if needed)

Fresh dill for garnish

Instructions:

Lay out the tortillas and spread a layer of cream cheese on each.

Place smoked salmon and avocado slices on the tortillas.

Garnish with fresh dill.

Roll the tortillas into wraps and slice in half.

Nutritional Benefits:

Salmon provides omega-3 fatty acids and protein. Avocado adds healthy fats and creaminess, while whole-grain tortillas offer fiber.

Blueberry Almond Smoothie

Ingredients (for 2 servings):

1 cup blueberries (fresh or frozen)

1 banana

1 cup almond milk (or lactose-free milk)

2 tablespoons almond butter

1 tablespoon chia seeds

Ice cubes (optional)

Instructions:

In a blender, combine blueberries, banana, almond milk, almond butter, and chia seeds.

Add ice cubes if desired and blend until smooth.

Pour into glasses and serve immediately.

Nutritional Benefits:

Blueberries are rich in antioxidants, while almond butter provides healthy fats and protein. Chia seeds add fiber and omega-3 fatty acids.

Spinach and Mushroom Omelette

Ingredients (for 2 servings):

4 eggs

1 cup fresh spinach, chopped

1/2 cup mushrooms, sliced

Salt and pepper to taste

1 tablespoon olive oil

Instructions:

In a bowl, whisk eggs and season with salt and pepper.

Heat olive oil in a pan over medium heat.

Add spinach and mushrooms to the pan and sauté until tender.

Pour the whisked eggs into the pan and cook until set.

Fold the omelette in half and serve.

Nutritional Benefits:

Eggs provide high-quality protein, while spinach and mushrooms offer vitamins and minerals. Olive oil adds healthy fats.

Sweet Potato Breakfast Hash

Ingredients (for 2 servings):

2 medium sweet potatoes, peeled and diced

1 bell pepper, diced

1/2 onion, diced

2 tablespoons olive oil

1 teaspoon paprika

Salt and pepper to taste

Poached eggs for topping

Instructions:

In a skillet, heat olive oil over medium heat.

Add diced sweet potatoes, bell pepper, and onion to the skillet.

Season with paprika, salt, and pepper. Cook until vegetables are tender.

Divide into two plates and top with poached eggs.

Nutritional Benefits:

Sweet potatoes are rich in vitamins and fiber. Bell peppers add color and vitamin C, while poached eggs provide protein and healthy fats.

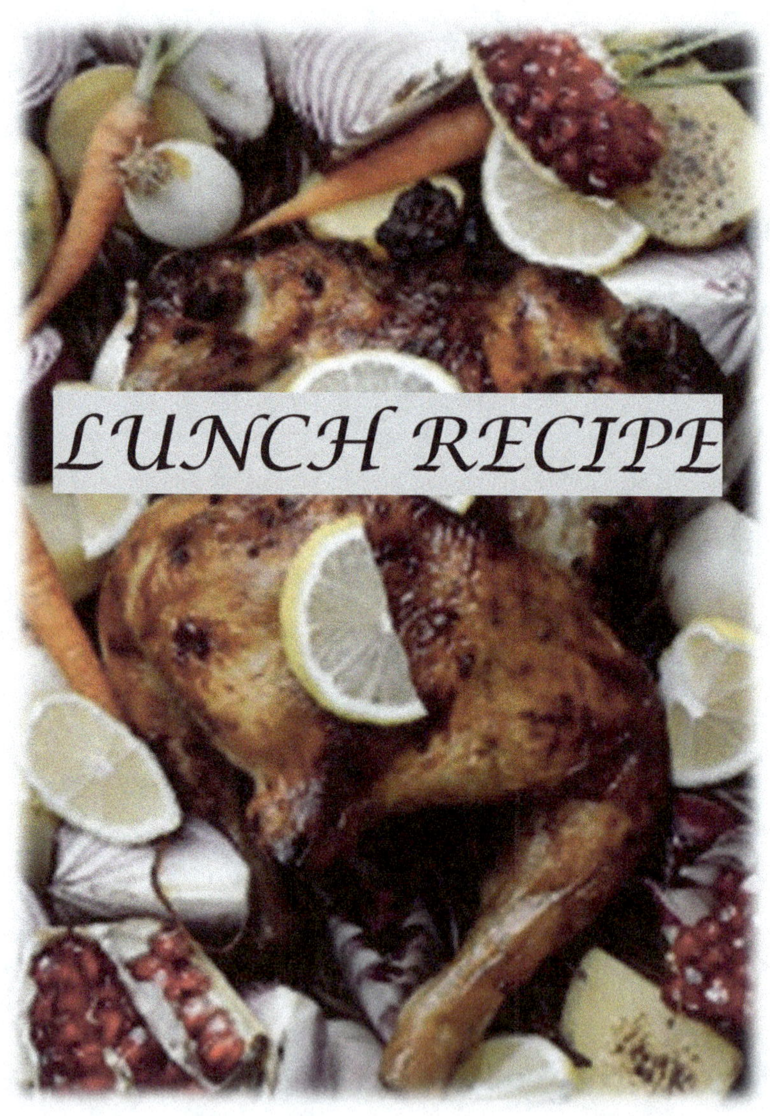

LUNCH RECIPE

Grilled Chicken and Vegetable Quinoa Bowl

Ingredients (for 2 servings):

1 cup cooked quinoa

2 boneless, skinless chicken breasts

1 zucchini, sliced

1 red bell pepper, sliced

1 tablespoon olive oil

Salt and pepper to taste

Fresh lemon juice for drizzling

Instructions:

Season chicken breasts with salt and pepper.

Heat olive oil in a grill pan over medium-high heat.

Grill chicken for 6-8 minutes per side or until cooked through.

In the same pan, grill zucchini and bell pepper until tender.

Slice chicken and serve over quinoa with grilled vegetables.

Drizzle with fresh lemon juice before serving.

Nutritional Benefits:

Quinoa provides protein and fiber, while grilled chicken offers lean protein. Zucchini and bell peppers add vitamins and antioxidants.

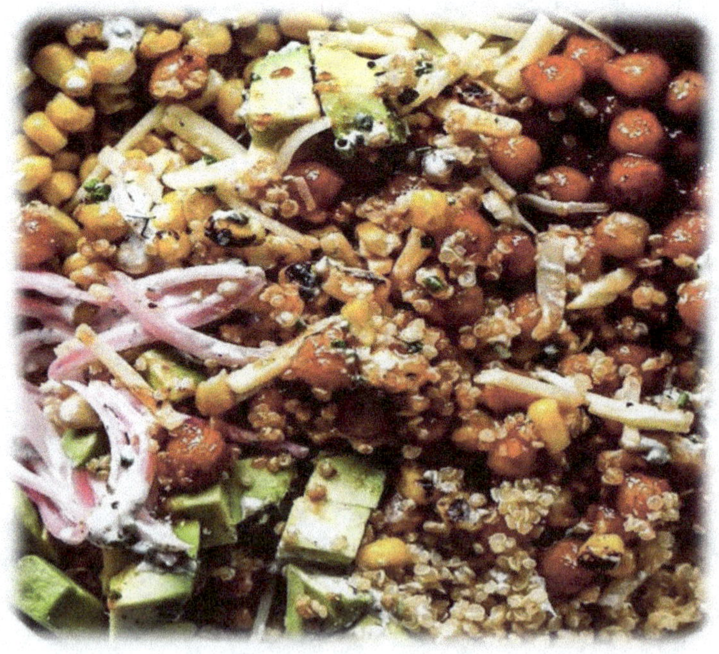

Salmon and Avocado Salad

Ingredients (for 2 servings):

2 salmon fillets

4 cups mixed salad greens

1 cucumber, sliced

1 avocado, diced

1/4 cup cherry tomatoes, halved

2 tablespoons olive oil

Balsamic vinaigrette for dressing

Instructions:

Season salmon fillets with salt and pepper.

In a pan, heat olive oil over medium-high heat and cook salmon for 4-5 minutes per side.

In a large bowl, toss salad greens, cucumber, avocado, and cherry tomatoes.

Top the salad with cooked salmon.

Drizzle with balsamic vinaigrette before serving.

Salmon provides omega-3 fatty acids and protein. Avocado adds healthy fats, and the salad greens offer vitamins and fiber.

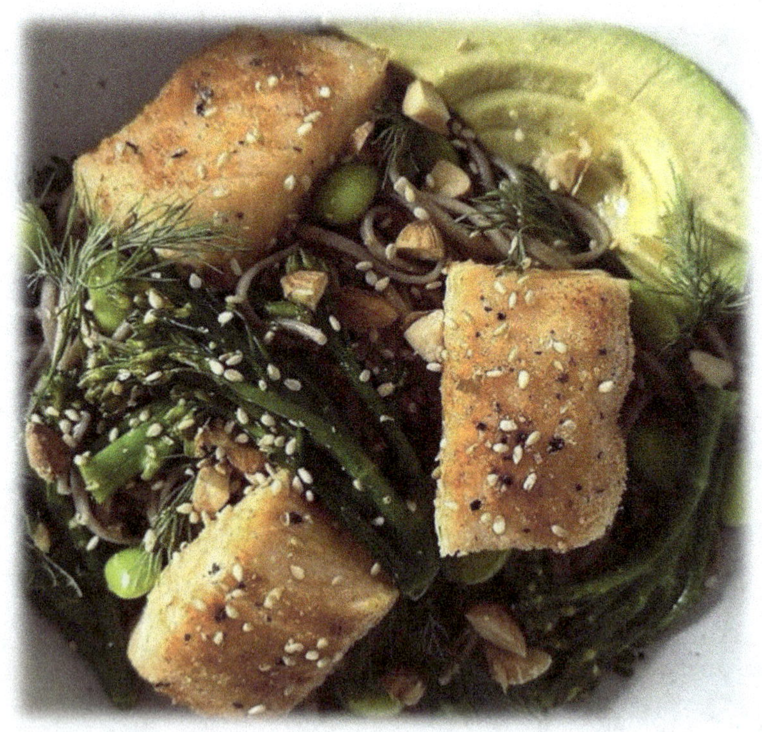

Turkey and Vegetable Stir-Fry

Ingredients (for 2 servings):

1/2-pound ground turkey

1 cup broccoli florets

1 carrot, julienned

1 bell pepper, sliced

2 tablespoons soy sauce (low sodium)

1 tablespoon sesame oil

1 tablespoon grated ginger

2 cups cooked brown rice

Instructions:

In a wok or large pan, brown ground turkey over medium heat.

Add broccoli, carrot, and bell pepper to the wok and stir-fry until vegetables are tender.

In a small bowl, mix soy sauce, sesame oil, and grated ginger.

Pour the sauce over the turkey and vegetables, stirring to coat.

Serve the stir-fry over cooked brown rice.

Nutritional Benefits:

Turkey provides lean protein, and vegetables offer vitamins and fiber. Brown rice adds complex carbohydrates.

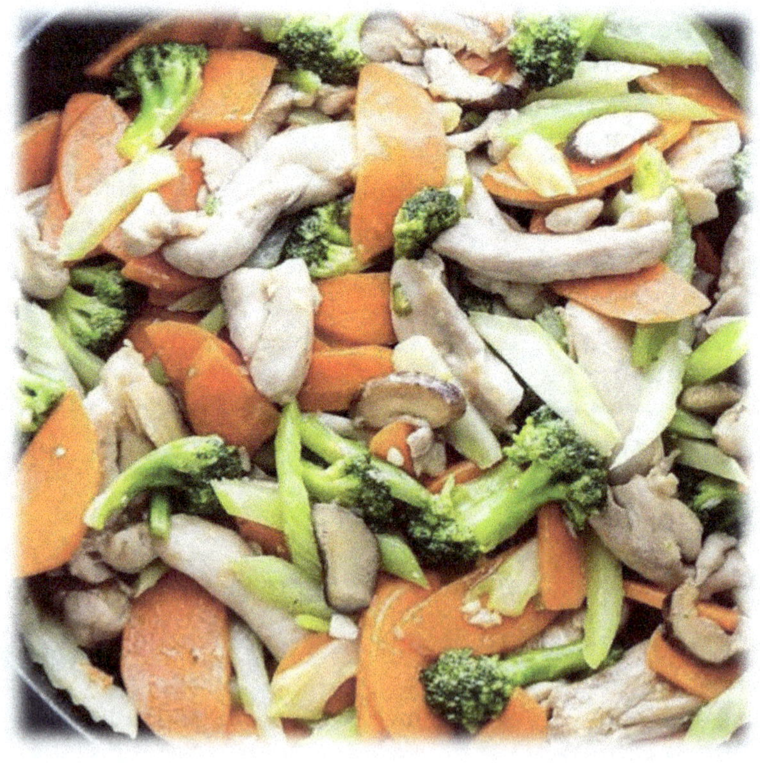

Lentil and Vegetable Soup

Ingredients (for 2 servings):

1 cup dried green lentils

1 onion, chopped

2 carrots, diced

2 celery stalks, chopped

3 cloves garlic, minced

4 cups vegetable broth (low sodium)

1 teaspoon cumin

Salt and pepper to taste

Fresh parsley for garnish

Instructions:

Rinse lentils and combine with chopped vegetables, garlic, and vegetable broth in a pot.

Bring to a boil, then reduce heat and simmer for 25-30 minutes or until lentils are tender.

Season with cumin, salt, and pepper.

Garnish with fresh parsley before serving.

Nutritional Benefits:

Lentils are a good source of plant-based protein and fiber. Vegetables add vitamins and minerals, creating a nourishing soup.

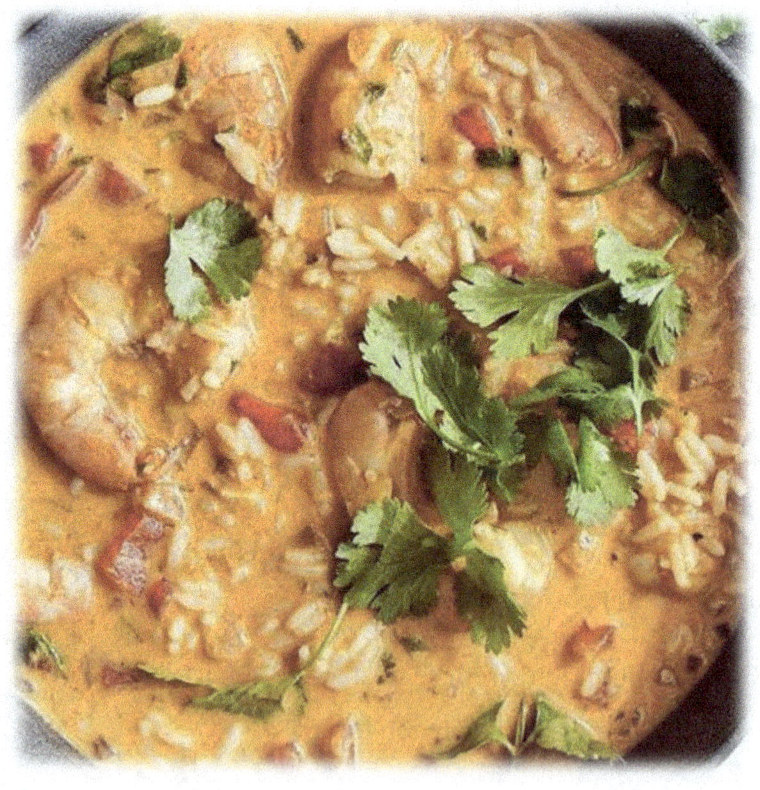

Shrimp and Spinach Salad with Lemon Vinaigrette

Ingredients (for 2 servings):

1/2-pound shrimp, peeled and deveined

4 cups fresh spinach

1 cup cherry tomatoes, halved

1/4 cup feta cheese, crumbled

2 tablespoons olive oil

Juice of 1 lemon

Salt and pepper to taste

Instructions:

Season shrimp with salt and pepper.

In a pan, heat olive oil over medium-high heat and cook shrimp for 2-3 minutes per side or until opaque.

In a large bowl, combine fresh spinach, cherry tomatoes, and crumbled feta.

Top the salad with cooked shrimp.

Whisk together lemon juice, olive oil, salt, and pepper. Drizzle over the salad before serving.

Nutritional Benefits:

Shrimp provides protein and omega-3 fatty acids. Spinach is rich in vitamins, and feta adds a touch of creaminess.

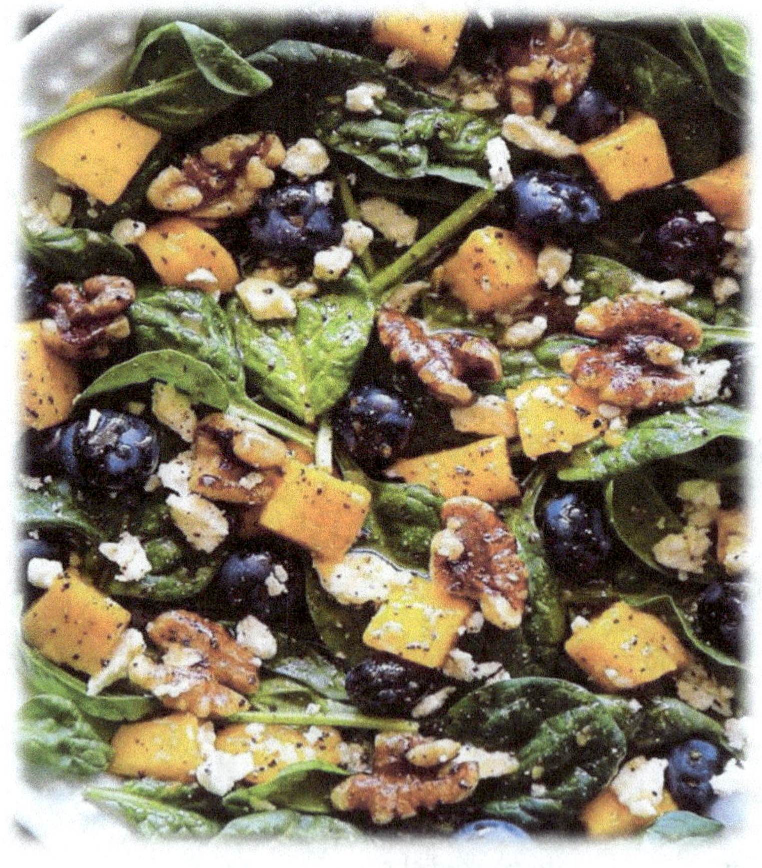

Chicken and Vegetable Wrap with Hummus

Ingredients (for 2 servings):

2 whole-grain wraps

1 grilled chicken breast, sliced

1 cup mixed salad greens

1 cucumber, julienned

1/4 cup hummus

Cherry tomatoes for garnish

Instructions:

Lay out the wraps and spread hummus evenly on each.

Place sliced grilled chicken, mixed salad greens, and julienned cucumber on the wraps.

Garnish with cherry tomatoes.

Roll the wraps and slice in half.

Whole-grain wraps provide fiber, while grilled chicken offers lean protein. Hummus adds a creamy texture and additional protein.

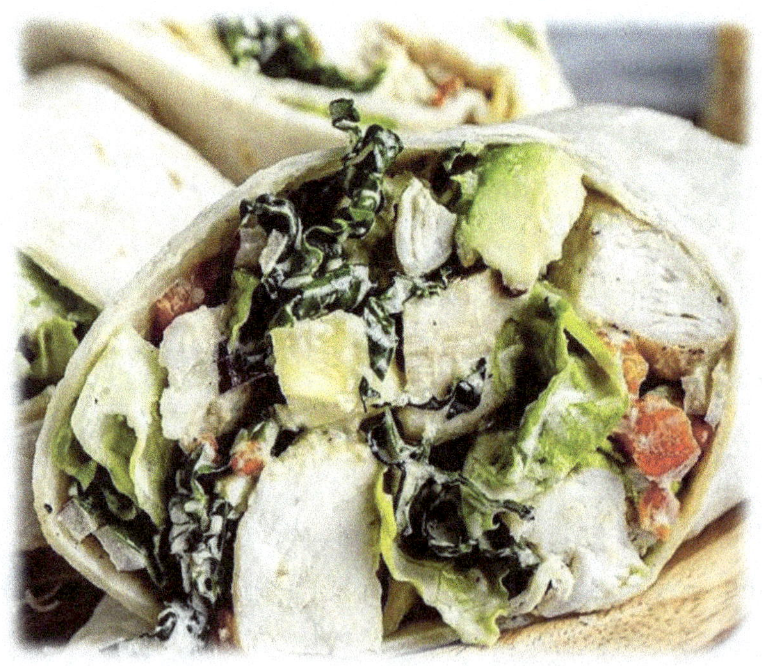

Sweet Potato and Turkey Skillet

Ingredients (for 2 servings):

1/2-pound ground turkey

2 medium sweet potatoes, peeled and diced

1 bell pepper, diced

1 teaspoon smoked paprika

Salt and pepper to taste

2 tablespoons olive oil

Fresh cilantro for garnish

Instructions:

In a skillet, heat olive oil over medium heat. Brown ground turkey until cooked through.

Add diced sweet potatoes and bell pepper to the skillet. Cook until sweet potatoes are tender.

Season with smoked paprika, salt, and pepper.

Garnish with fresh cilantro before serving.

Sweet potatoes provide vitamins and fiber, while ground turkey offers lean protein. Bell peppers add color and antioxidants.

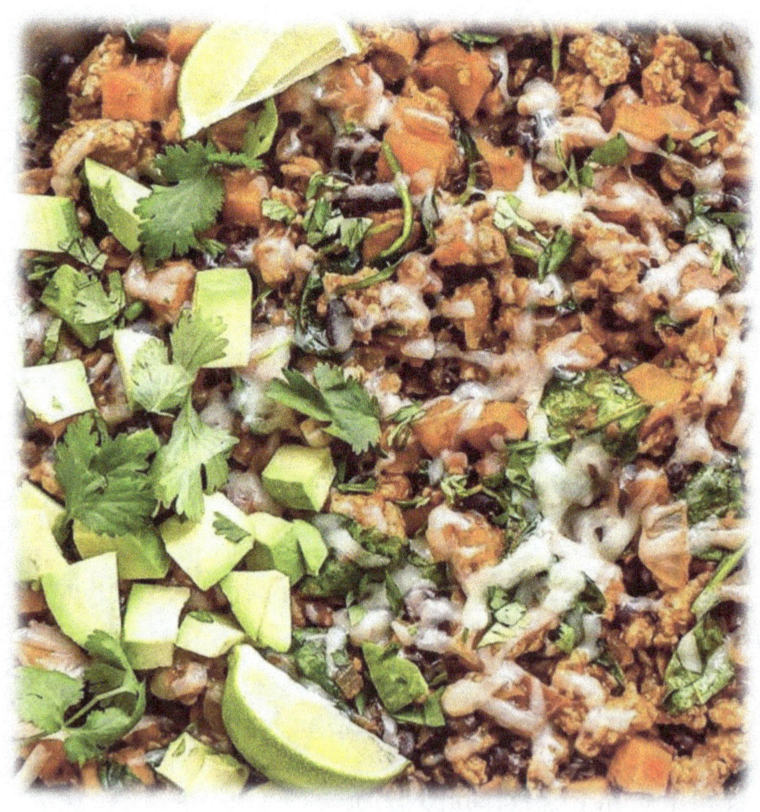

Miso-Ginger Tofu Stir-Fry

Ingredients (for 2 servings):

1 cup extra-firm tofu, cubed

2 cups broccoli florets

1 carrot, julienned

2 tablespoons miso paste

1 tablespoon soy sauce (low sodium)

1 tablespoon grated ginger

1 tablespoon sesame oil

2 cups cooked brown rice

Instructions:

In a wok or large pan, heat sesame oil over medium-high heat.

Add cubed tofu and stir-fry until golden brown.

Add broccoli and julienned carrot to the wok and stir-fry until vegetables are tender.

In a small bowl, mix miso paste, soy sauce, and grated ginger. Pour over the tofu and vegetables.

Serve the stir-fry over cooked brown rice.

Nutritional Benefits:

Tofu provides plant-based protein, and vegetables offer vitamins and fiber. Miso adds a rich umami flavor without excessive sodium.

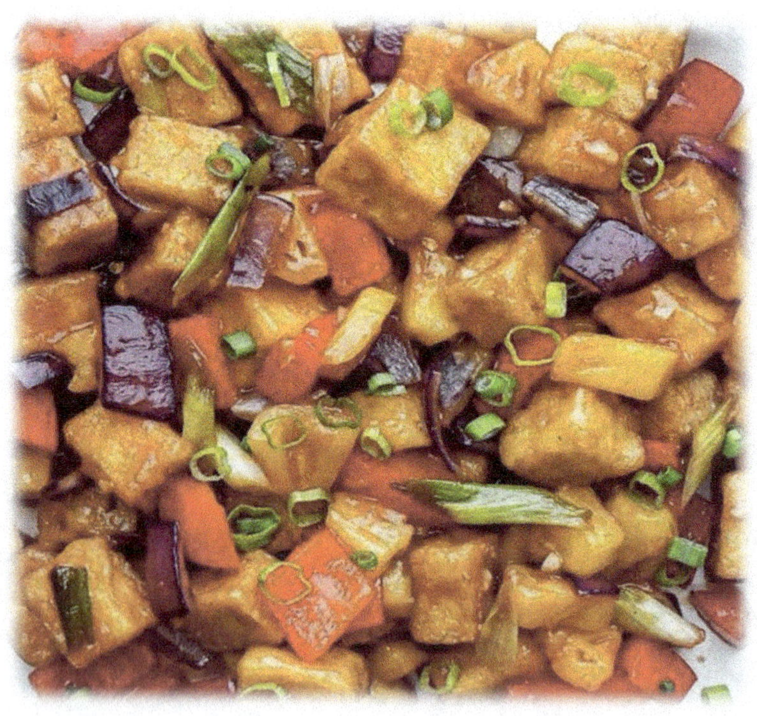

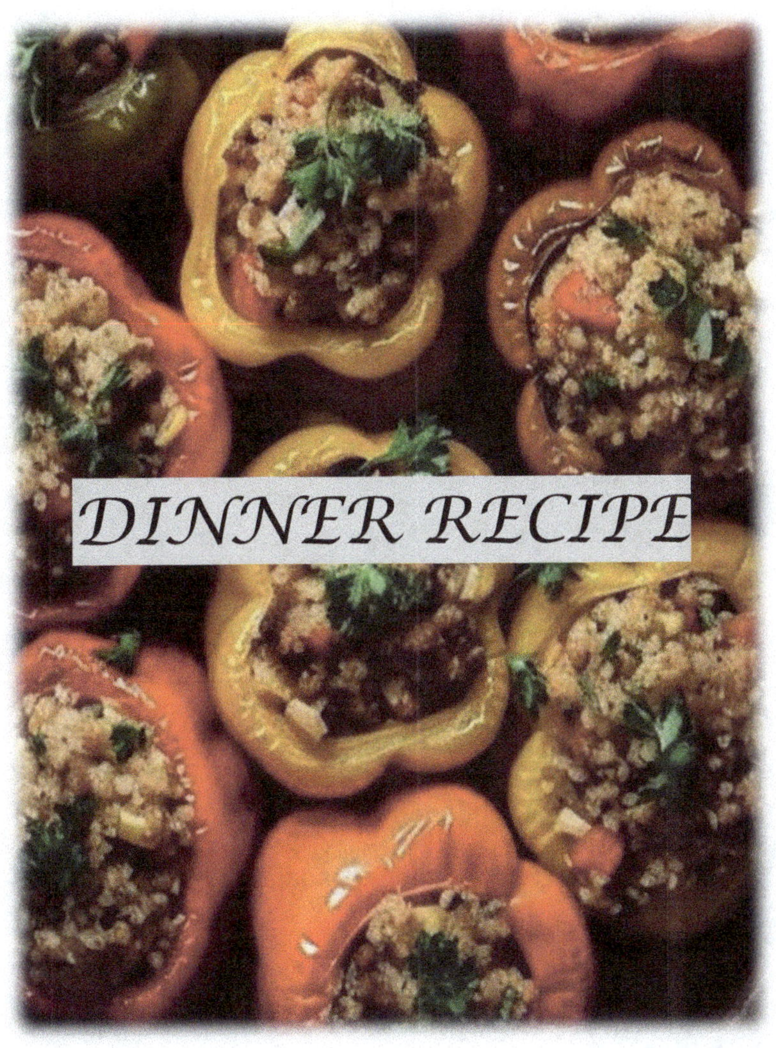
DINNER RECIPE

Quinoa and Vegetable Stuffed Peppers

Ingredients (for 2 servings):

1 cup cooked quinoa

2 bell peppers, halved and seeds removed

1 cup black beans, cooked and drained

1 cup corn kernels (fresh or frozen)

1 cup cherry tomatoes, halved

1 teaspoon cumin

Salt and pepper to taste

Fresh cilantro for garnish

Instructions:

Preheat the oven to 375°F (190°C).

In a bowl, combine cooked quinoa, black beans, corn, cherry tomatoes, cumin, salt, and pepper.

Stuff the bell peppers with the quinoa mixture.

Bake for 25-30 minutes or until peppers are tender.

Garnish with fresh cilantro before serving.

Nutritional Benefits:

Quinoa provides protein and fiber, black beans offer plant-based protein, and bell peppers add vitamins.

Baked Lemon Herb Chicken

Ingredients (for 2 servings):

2 boneless, skinless chicken breasts

2 tablespoons olive oil

1 lemon, juiced

2 cloves garlic, minced

1 teaspoon dried thyme

Salt and pepper to taste

Fresh parsley for garnish

Instructions:

Preheat the oven to 375°F (190°C).

In a bowl, mix olive oil, lemon juice, minced garlic, dried thyme, salt, and pepper.

Marinate chicken breasts in the mixture for 30 minutes.

Place chicken in a baking dish and bake for 25-30 minutes or until cooked through.

Garnish with fresh parsley before serving.

Nutritional Benefits:

Chicken provides lean protein, while olive oil adds healthy fats. Lemon and thyme contribute flavor without excessive seasoning.

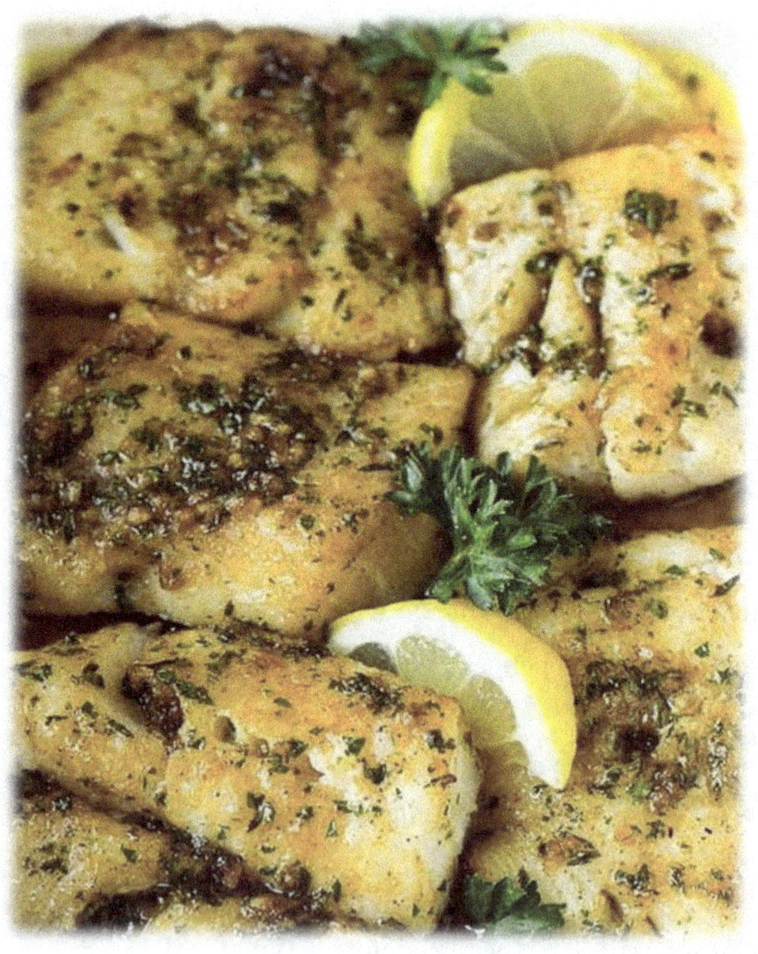

Salmon and Asparagus Foil Packets

Ingredients (for 2 servings):

2 salmon fillets

1 bunch asparagus, trimmed

2 tablespoons olive oil

1 lemon, sliced

2 cloves garlic, minced

Salt and pepper to taste

Instructions:

Preheat the oven to 400°F (200°C).

Place each salmon fillet on a piece of foil.

Arrange asparagus around the salmon, drizzle with olive oil, and sprinkle minced garlic.

Season with salt and pepper, and place lemon slices on top.

Fold the foil to create packets and bake for 20 minutes or until salmon is cooked through.

Nutritional Benefits:

Salmon provides omega-3 fatty acids and protein, while asparagus adds vitamins and fiber.

Turkey and Vegetable Quinoa Stir-Fry

Ingredients (for 2 servings):

1/2-pound ground turkey

1 cup broccoli florets

1 bell pepper, sliced

1 carrot, julienned

2 cups cooked quinoa

2 tablespoons soy sauce (low sodium)

1 tablespoon sesame oil

1 tablespoon grated ginger

Instructions:

In a wok or large pan, brown ground turkey over medium heat.

Add broccoli, bell pepper, and julienned carrot. Stir-fry until vegetables are tender.

Stir in cooked quinoa, soy sauce, sesame oil, and grated ginger.

Cook until heated through and serve.

Nutritional Benefits:

Turkey provides lean protein, and vegetables offer vitamins and fiber. Quinoa adds protein and complex carbohydrates.

Lemon Garlic Shrimp Pasta

Ingredients (for 2 servings):

8 oz whole-grain or gluten-free spaghetti

1/2-pound shrimp, peeled and deveined

2 tablespoons olive oil

3 cloves garlic, minced

1 lemon, zested and juiced

Fresh parsley for garnish

Salt and pepper to taste

Instructions:

Cook pasta according to package instructions.

In a pan, heat olive oil over medium heat. Add minced garlic and sauté until fragrant.

Add shrimp to the pan and cook until opaque.

Toss cooked pasta with shrimp, lemon zest, and lemon juice.

Garnish with fresh parsley before serving.

Nutritional Benefits:

Shrimp provides protein and omega-3 fatty acids. Whole-grain pasta adds fiber, and lemon offers a burst of flavor.

Vegetarian Chickpea and Spinach Curry

Ingredients (for 2 servings):

1 can chickpeas, drained and rinsed

1 onion, chopped

2 tomatoes, diced

2 cups fresh spinach

1 can coconut milk

2 tablespoons curry powder

1 tablespoon olive oil

Salt and pepper to taste

Basmati rice for serving

Instructions:

In a pan, heat olive oil over medium heat. Sauté chopped onion until softened.

Add diced tomatoes and chickpeas to the pan, stirring to combine.

Pour in coconut milk and add curry powder. Simmer for 15 minutes.

Stir in fresh spinach until wilted.

Season with salt and pepper and serve over basmati rice.

Nutritional Benefits:

Chickpeas provide plant-based protein and fiber. Spinach adds vitamins, and coconut milk contributes healthy fats.

Eggplant and Tomato Lentil Soup

Ingredients (for 2 servings):

1 cup dried green lentils

1 eggplant, diced

1 can diced tomatoes

1 onion, chopped

2 carrots, diced

3 cloves garlic, minced

4 cups vegetable broth (low sodium)

1 teaspoon cumin

Salt and pepper to taste

Fresh cilantro for garnish

Instructions:

Rinse lentils and combine with diced eggplant, diced tomatoes, chopped onion, carrots, minced garlic, and vegetable broth in a pot.

Bring to a boil, then reduce heat and simmer for 25-30 minutes or until lentils are tender.

Season with cumin, salt, and pepper.

Garnish with fresh cilantro before serving.

Nutritional Benefits:

Lentils provide plant-based protein and fiber. Eggplant and tomatoes add vitamins and antioxidants.

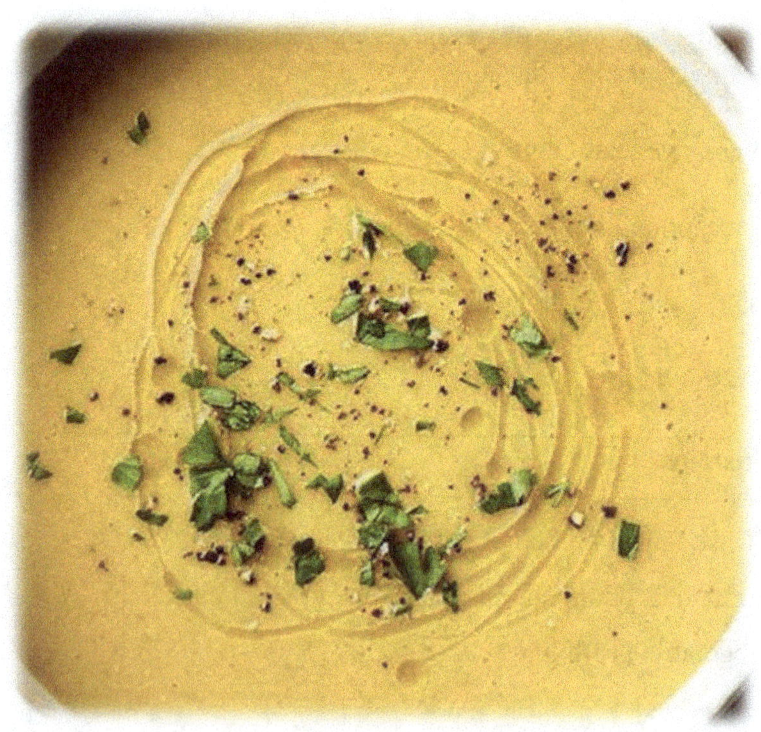

Miso-Glazed Baked Tofu

Ingredients (for 2 servings):

1 cup extra-firm tofu, cubed

2 tablespoons miso paste

1 tablespoon soy sauce (low sodium)

1 tablespoon maple syrup

1 tablespoon sesame oil

1 teaspoon grated ginger

Sesame seeds for garnish

Green onions for garnish

Instructions:

Preheat the oven to 400°F (200°C).

In a bowl, whisk together miso paste, soy sauce, maple syrup, sesame oil, and grated ginger.

Toss tofu cubes in the miso mixture until well coated.

Place tofu on a baking sheet and bake for 25-30 minutes or until golden brown.

Garnish with sesame seeds and green onions before serving.

Nutritional Benefits:

Tofu provides plant-based protein. Miso adds rich umami flavor, and sesame oil contributes healthy fats.

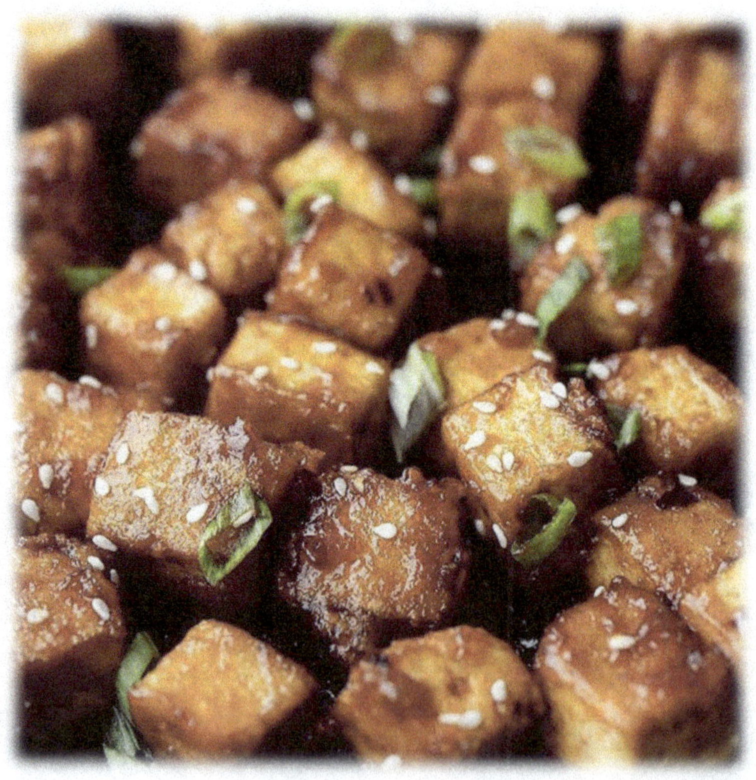

Chicken and Vegetable Skewers with Quinoa

Ingredients (for 2 servings):

2 boneless, skinless chicken breasts, cut into cubes

1 zucchini, sliced

1 bell pepper, diced

1 cup cherry tomatoes

2 tablespoons olive oil

1 lemon, juiced

1 teaspoon dried oregano

Salt and pepper to taste

1 cup cooked quinoa for serving

Instructions:

Preheat the grill or grill pan.

Thread chicken cubes, zucchini slices, bell pepper pieces, and cherry tomatoes onto skewers.

In a bowl, mix olive oil, lemon juice, dried oregano, salt, and pepper.

Brush the skewers with the olive oil mixture and grill for 10-12 minutes or until chicken is cooked through.

Serve over cooked quinoa.

Nutritional Benefits:

Chicken provides lean protein, and vegetables offer vitamins and fiber. Quinoa adds protein and complex carbohydrates.

Vegetable and Tofu Stir-Fried Rice

Ingredients (for 2 servings):

2 cups cooked brown rice

1 cup extra-firm tofu, cubed

1 cup broccoli florets

1 carrot, julienned

1/2 cup frozen peas

2 tablespoons soy sauce (low sodium)

1 tablespoon sesame oil

1 tablespoon grated ginger

2 green onions, sliced

Instructions:

In a wok or large pan, heat sesame oil over medium-high heat.

Add tofu cubes and stir-fry until golden brown.

Add broccoli, julienned carrot, and frozen peas. Stir-fry until vegetables are tender.

Stir in cooked brown rice, soy sauce, and grated ginger.

Cook until heated through and garnish with sliced green onions.

Nutritional Benefits:

Tofu provides plant-based protein, and brown rice adds fiber. Vegetables offer vitamins and minerals, creating a balanced and flavorful dish.

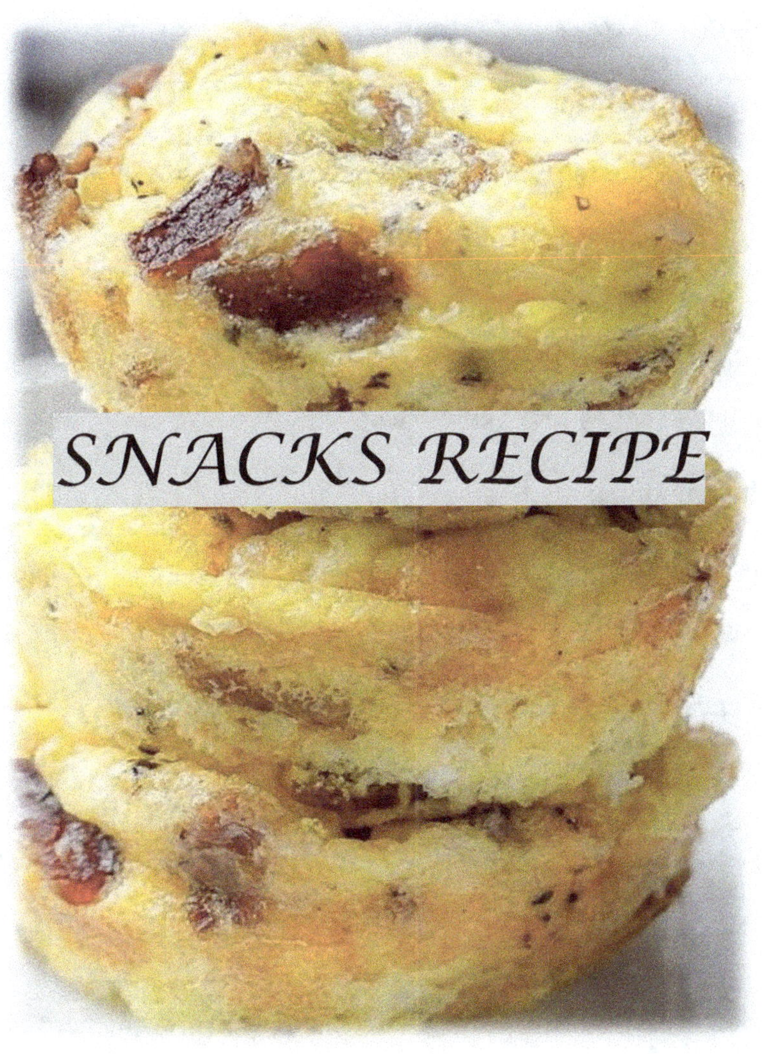
SNACKS RECIPE

Greek Yogurt Parfait with Berries

Ingredients (for 2 servings):

1 cup Greek yogurt (lactose-free if needed)

1 cup mixed berries (blueberries, raspberries, strawberries)

1/4 cup granola

1 tablespoon honey (optional)

Instructions:

In two glasses or bowls, layer Greek yogurt, mixed berries, and granola.

Repeat the layers.

Drizzle with honey if desired.

Serve chilled.

Nutritional Benefits:

Greek yogurt provides probiotics and protein, while berries offer antioxidants. Granola adds crunch and additional fiber.

Hummus and Veggie Sticks

Ingredients (for 2 servings):

1 cup hummus

1 cucumber, cut into sticks

2 carrots, cut into sticks

1 bell pepper, sliced

Instructions:

Arrange veggie sticks on a plate.

Serve with hummus for dipping.

Enjoy as a crunchy and satisfying snack.

Nutritional Benefits:

Hummus provides protein and healthy fats, while veggies offer vitamins and fiber.

Almond Butter Banana Bites

Ingredients (for 2 servings):

2 bananas, sliced

4 tablespoons almond butter

2 tablespoons chia seeds

1 tablespoon shredded coconut (optional)

Instructions:

Spread almond butter on banana slices.

Sprinkle chia seeds and shredded coconut on top.

Arrange on a plate and serve.

Nutritional Benefits:

Bananas offer potassium, while almond butter provides healthy fats and protein. Chia seeds add omega-3 fatty acids.

Rice Cake with Avocado and Cherry Tomatoes

Ingredients (for 2 servings):

2 rice cakes

1 avocado, mashed

1 cup cherry tomatoes, halved

Salt and pepper to taste

Red pepper flakes for optional heat

Instructions:

Spread mashed avocado on rice cakes.

Top with halved cherry tomatoes.

Season with salt, pepper, and red pepper flakes if desired.

Serve as a quick and tasty snack.

Nutritional Benefits:

Rice cakes provide a light base, while avocado offers
healthy fats and vitamins. Cherry tomatoes add freshness.

Smoothie Bowl with Spinach and Pineapple

Ingredients (for 2 servings):

2 cups fresh spinach

1 cup frozen pineapple chunks

1 banana

1/2 cup coconut water

Toppings: sliced strawberries, chia seeds

Instructions:

Blend spinach, frozen pineapple, banana, and coconut water until smooth.

Pour into bowls and top with sliced strawberries and chia seeds.

Enjoy this nutrient-packed and refreshing snack.

Nutritional Benefits:

Spinach provides vitamins and minerals, while pineapple adds natural sweetness. Chia seeds contribute omega-3 fatty acids.

Cottage Cheese and Pineapple Cups

Ingredients (for 2 servings):

1 cup low-fat cottage cheese

1 cup fresh pineapple chunks

2 tablespoons chopped mint (optional)

Instructions:

In two small bowls, scoop cottage cheese.

Top with fresh pineapple chunks.

Garnish with chopped mint if desired.

Serve chilled.

Nutritional Benefits:

Cottage cheese is a good source of protein, while pineapple offers vitamins and natural sweetness.

Baked Sweet Potato Chips

Ingredients (for 2 servings):

2 medium sweet potatoes, peeled and thinly sliced

2 tablespoons olive oil

1 teaspoon paprika

1/2 teaspoon garlic powder

Salt and pepper to taste

Instructions:

Preheat the oven to 375°F (190°C).

Toss sweet potato slices with olive oil, paprika, garlic powder, salt, and pepper.

Arrange in a single layer on a baking sheet.

Bake for 20-25 minutes or until crispy.

Allow to cool before serving.

Nutritional Benefits:

Sweet potatoes provide vitamins and fiber. Baking instead of frying makes these chips a healthier snack.

Chia Seed Pudding with Mango

Ingredients (for 2 servings):

1/4 cup chia seeds

1 cup almond milk (or lactose-free milk)

1 teaspoon vanilla extract

1 tablespoon maple syrup

1 mango, diced

Instructions:

In a bowl, mix chia seeds, almond milk, vanilla extract, and maple syrup.

Refrigerate for at least 4 hours or overnight.

Divide into two servings and top with diced mango before serving.

Nutritional Benefits:

Chia seeds provide omega-3 fatty acids and fiber. Almond milk adds creaminess, and mango offers natural sweetness.

Cherry Almond Energy Bites

Ingredients (for 2 servings):

1 cup dried cherries

1/2 cup almonds

1/4 cup rolled oats

1 tablespoon honey

1/2 teaspoon vanilla extract

Instructions:

In a food processor, blend dried cherries, almonds, rolled oats, honey, and vanilla extract until well combined.

Roll the mixture into small energy bites.

Refrigerate for at least 30 minutes before serving.

Nutritional Benefits:

Cherries provide antioxidants, while almonds offer healthy fats and protein. Oats add fiber and energy.

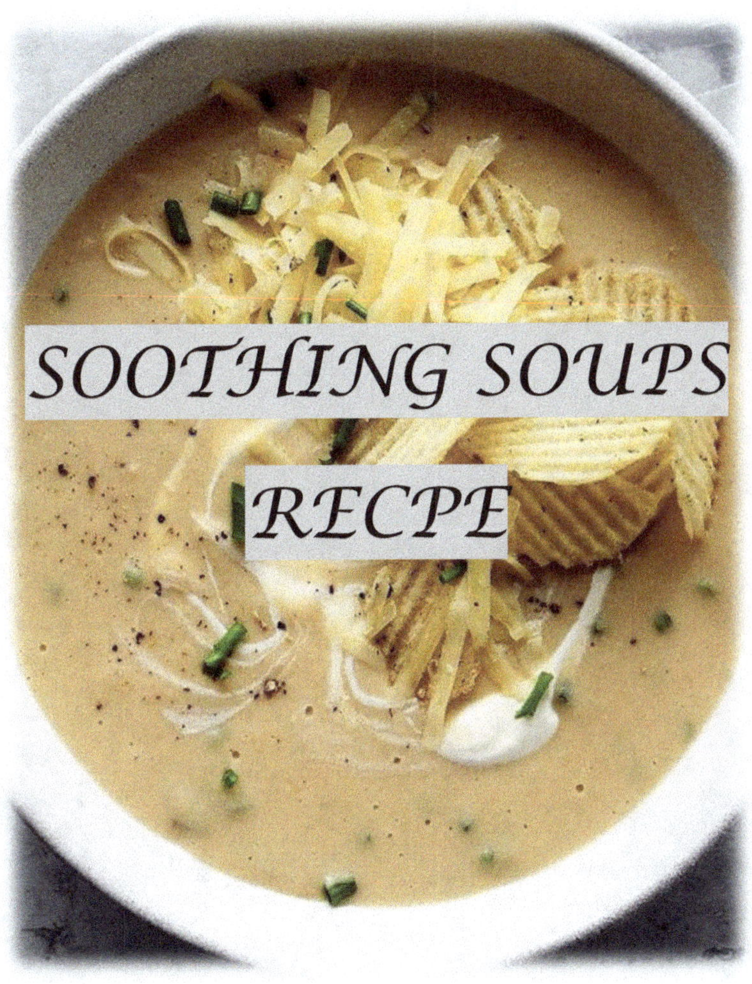
SOOTHING SOUPS
RECPE

Carrot and Ginger Soup

Ingredients (for 2 servings):

4 large carrots, peeled and chopped

1 onion, chopped

2 cloves garlic, minced

1 tablespoon fresh ginger, grated

4 cups vegetable broth (low sodium)

1 tablespoon olive oil

Salt and pepper to taste

Fresh cilantro for garnish (optional)

Instructions:

In a pot, heat olive oil over medium heat. Add chopped onion, garlic, and grated ginger. Sauté until fragrant.

Add chopped carrots and continue to sauté for 5 minutes.

Pour in vegetable broth, bring to a boil, then simmer until carrots are tender.

Use an immersion blender to puree the soup until smooth.

Season with salt and pepper, and garnish with fresh cilantro if desired.

Nutritional Benefits:

Carrots are rich in beta-carotene, while ginger provides anti-inflammatory properties. This soup is easy to digest and soothing on the stomach.

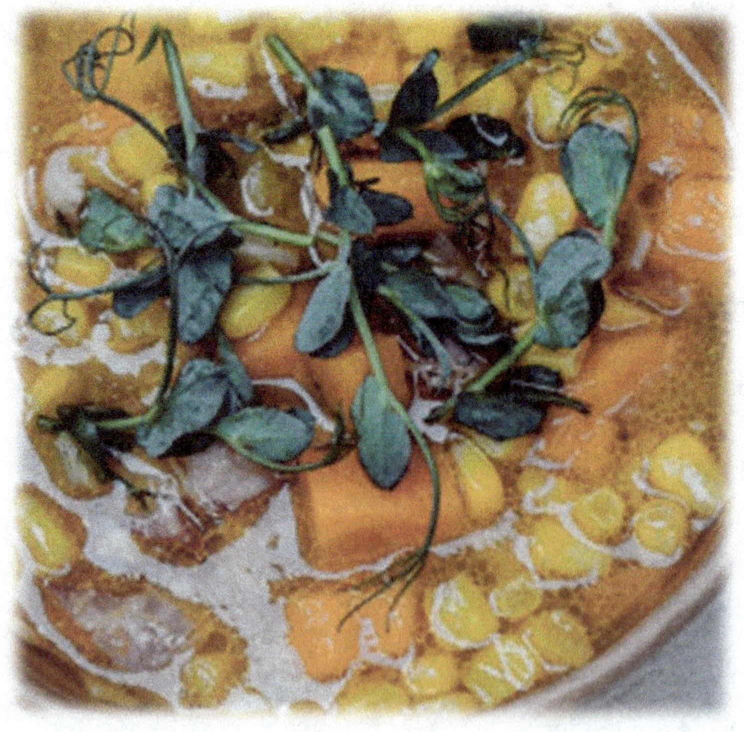

Minty Pea Soup

Ingredients (for 2 servings):

2 cups frozen peas

1 onion, chopped

2 cups vegetable broth (low sodium)

1 tablespoon olive oil

Fresh mint leaves for flavor

Salt and pepper to taste

Lemon wedges for serving (optional)

Instructions:

In a pot, heat olive oil over medium heat. Add chopped onion and sauté until softened.

Add frozen peas and vegetable broth. Bring to a boil, then simmer until peas are tender.

Remove from heat and blend the soup until smooth with an immersion blender.

Stir in fresh mint leaves and season with salt and pepper.

Serve with a squeeze of lemon if desired.

Nutritional Benefits:

Peas provide fiber and essential nutrients, while mint adds a refreshing flavor. This soup is gentle on the digestive system.

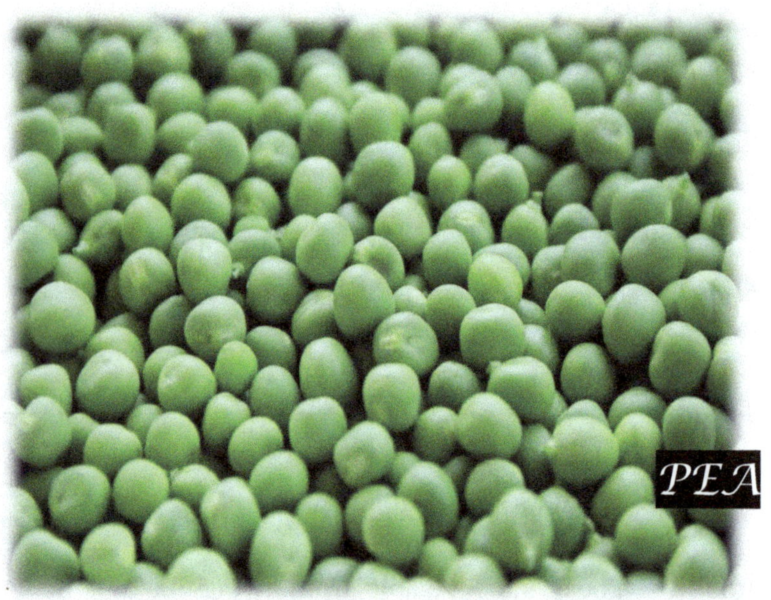

Butternut Squash and Apple Soup

Ingredients (for 2 servings):

2 cups butternut squash, peeled and diced

1 apple, peeled and chopped

1 onion, chopped

4 cups vegetable broth (low sodium)

1 tablespoon olive oil

1/2 teaspoon cinnamon

Salt and pepper to taste

Toasted pumpkin seeds for garnish (optional)

Instructions:

In a pot, heat olive oil over medium heat. Add chopped onion and sauté until translucent.

Add diced butternut squash and apple. Sauté for 5 minutes.

Pour in vegetable broth and bring to a boil. Simmer until vegetables are tender.

Use an immersion blender to puree the soup until smooth.

Season with cinnamon, salt, and pepper. Garnish with toasted pumpkin seeds if desired.

Nutritional Benefits:

Butternut squash is rich in vitamins, and apples add natural sweetness. This soup provides a comforting blend of flavors.

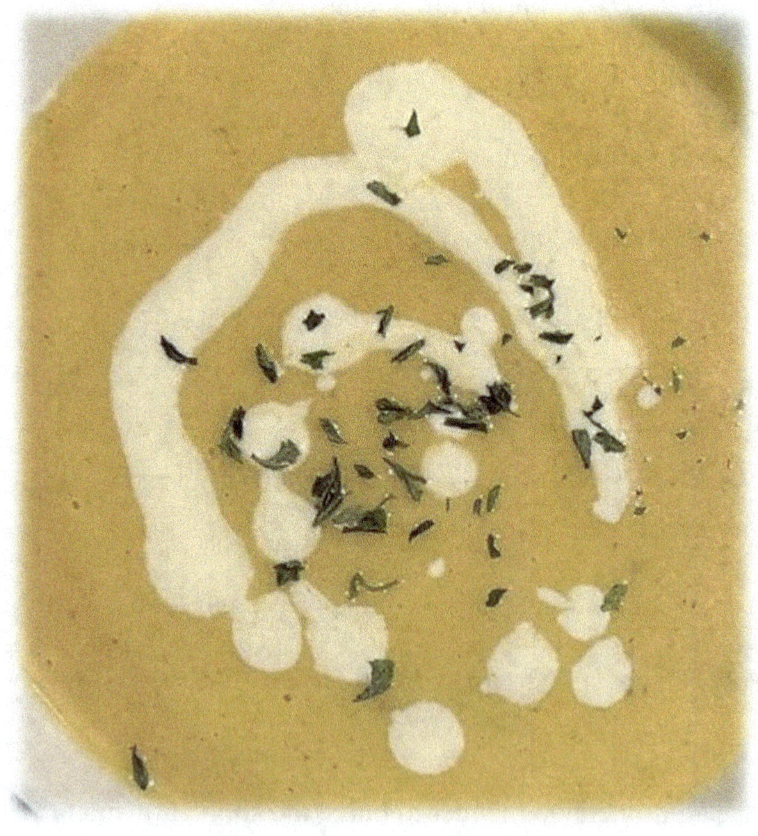

Quinoa and Kale Soup

Ingredients (for 2 servings):

1/2 cup quinoa, rinsed

1 cup kale, chopped

1 carrot, diced

1 celery stalk, diced

1 onion, chopped

4 cups vegetable broth (low sodium)

1 tablespoon olive oil

2 cloves garlic, minced

Salt and pepper to taste

Fresh parsley for garnish (optional)

Instructions:

In a pot, heat olive oil over medium heat. Add chopped onion and minced garlic. Sauté until fragrant.

Add diced carrot, celery, and kale. Sauté for 5 minutes.

Pour in vegetable broth and bring to a boil. Add rinsed quinoa and simmer until quinoa is cooked.

Season with salt and pepper. Garnish with fresh parsley if desired.

Nutritional Benefits:

Quinoa provides protein and fiber, while kale adds vitamins and minerals. This soup is a nourishing option for Crohn's disease.

Tomato Basil Soup

Ingredients (for 2 servings):

2 cups canned tomatoes

1 onion, chopped

2 cloves garlic, minced

4 cups vegetable broth (low sodium)

1/4 cup fresh basil leaves, chopped

1 tablespoon olive oil

Salt and pepper to taste

Grated Parmesan cheese for garnish (optional)

Instructions:

In a pot, heat olive oil over medium heat. Add chopped onion and minced garlic. Sauté until softened.

Add canned tomatoes and vegetable broth. Bring to a boil, then simmer for 15 minutes.

Use an immersion blender to puree the soup until smooth.

Stir in chopped basil and season with salt and pepper.

Garnish with grated Parmesan cheese if desired.

Nutritional Benefits:

Tomatoes provide lycopene, and basil adds a burst of flavor. This soup is gentle on the stomach and easy to digest.

Chicken and Rice Congee

Ingredients (for 2 servings):

1/2 cup white rice

2 cups chicken broth (low sodium)

1 cup cooked shredded chicken

1 inch ginger, grated

1 tablespoon soy sauce (low sodium)

Green onions for garnish

Sesame oil for drizzling (optional)

Instructions:

In a pot, combine white rice, chicken broth, grated ginger, and soy sauce. Bring to a simmer.

Cook until the rice is soft and the congee has a creamy consistency.

Stir in shredded chicken and cook until heated through.

Garnish with chopped green onions and drizzle with sesame oil if desired.

Congee is a gentle and easily digestible rice porridge. Chicken adds protein, and ginger provides anti-inflammatory properties.

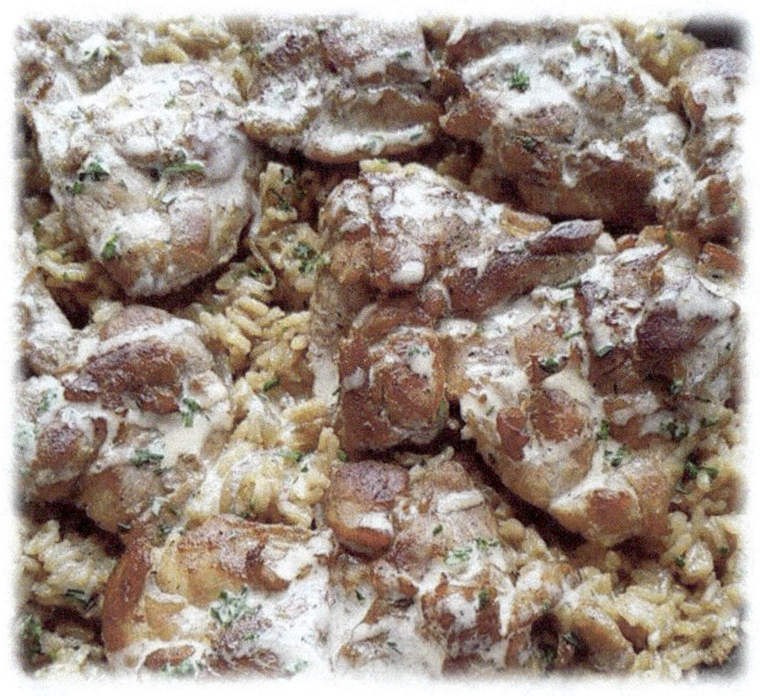

Lentil and Spinach Soup

Ingredients (for 2 servings):

1 cup dried green lentils

2 cups fresh spinach

1 carrot, diced

1 celery stalk, diced

1 onion, chopped

4 cups vegetable broth (low sodium)

1 tablespoon olive oil

2 cloves garlic, minced

1 teaspoon cumin

Salt and pepper to taste

Instructions:

Rinse lentils and set aside.

In a pot, heat olive oil over medium heat. Add chopped onion and minced garlic. Sauté until fragrant.

Add diced carrot, diced celery, and cumin. Sauté for 5 minutes.

Pour in vegetable broth and bring to a boil. Add rinsed lentils and simmer until lentils are tender.

Stir in fresh spinach until wilted. Season with salt and pepper.

Nutritional Benefits:

Lentils provide plant-based protein and fiber, while spinach adds vitamins and minerals. This soup is easy on the digestive system.

Zucchini and Basil Soup

Ingredients (for 2 servings):

2 medium zucchinis, diced

1 onion, chopped

2 cloves garlic, minced

4 cups vegetable broth (low sodium)

1/4 cup fresh basil leaves, chopped

1 tablespoon olive oil

Salt and pepper to taste

Greek yogurt for garnish (optional)

Instructions:

In a pot, heat olive oil over medium heat. Add chopped onion and minced garlic. Sauté until softened.

Add diced zucchinis and vegetable broth. Bring to a boil, then simmer until zucchinis are tender.

Use an immersion blender to puree the soup until smooth.

Stir in chopped basil and season with salt and pepper.

Garnish with a dollop of Greek yogurt if desired.

Nutritional Benefits:

Zucchinis provide vitamins, and basil adds a fresh flavor.

This soup is light and soothing on the digestive system.

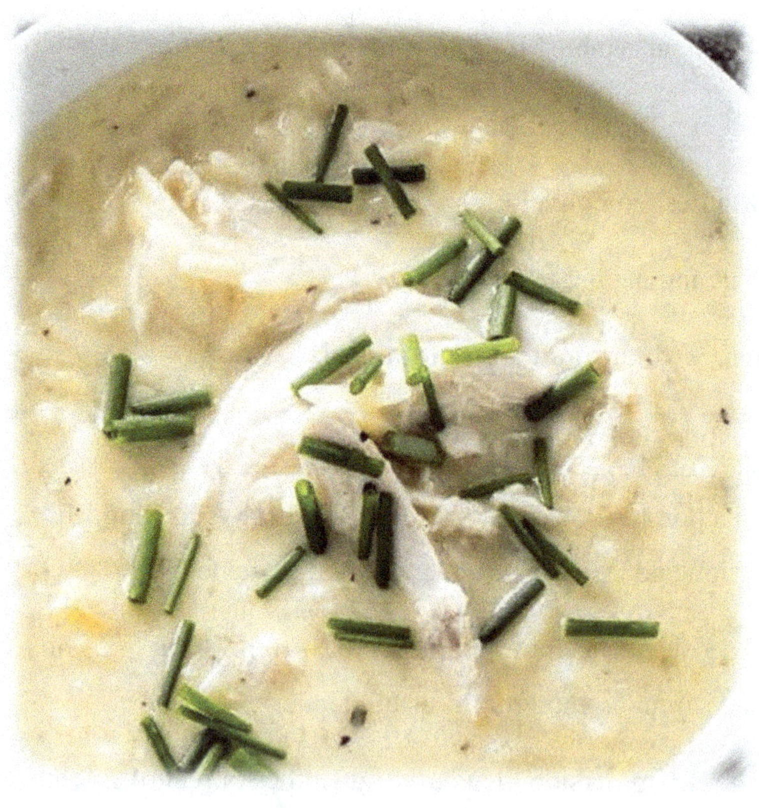

Creamy Spinach and Potato Soup

Ingredients (for 2 servings):

2 potatoes, peeled and diced

2 cups fresh spinach

1 onion, chopped

2 cups vegetable broth (low sodium)

1/2 cup unsweetened almond milk

1 tablespoon olive oil

Salt and pepper to taste

Nutmeg for optional flavor

Instructions:

In a pot, heat olive oil over medium heat. Add chopped onion and sauté until translucent.

Add diced potatoes and vegetable broth. Bring to a boil, then simmer until potatoes are soft.

Stir in fresh spinach until wilted.

Use an immersion blender to puree the soup until smooth.

Pour in almond milk, season with salt, pepper, and a pinch of nutmeg if desired.

Nutritional Benefits:

Potatoes provide carbohydrates, and spinach adds vitamins. Almond milk creates a creamy texture without dairy.

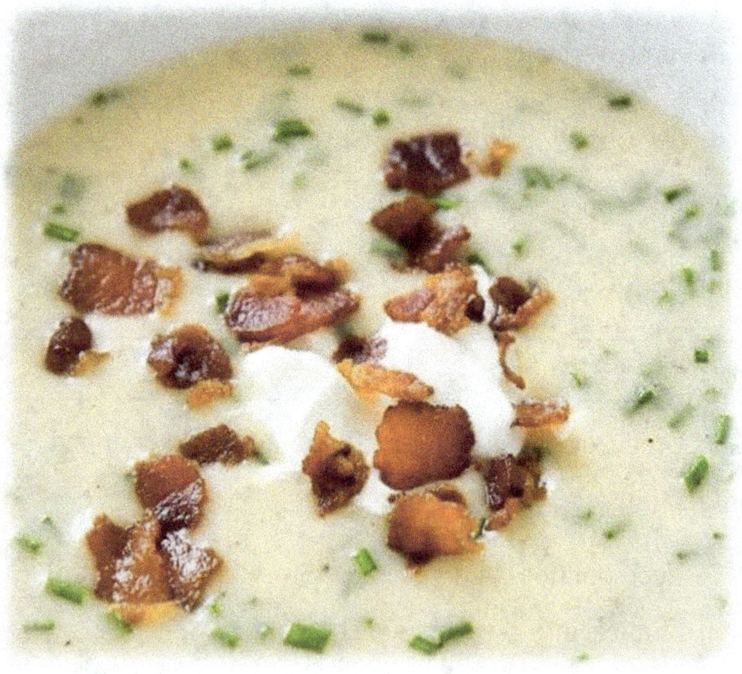

Turkey and Vegetable Soup

Ingredients (for 2 servings):

1/2-pound ground turkey

1 carrot, diced

1 celery stalk, diced

1 zucchini, diced

1 onion, chopped

4 cups chicken broth (low sodium)

1 tablespoon olive oil

2 cloves garlic, minced

1 teaspoon dried thyme

Salt and pepper to taste

Instructions:

In a pot, heat olive oil over medium heat. Add chopped onion and minced garlic. Sauté until softened.

Add ground turkey and cook until browned.

Add diced carrot, diced celery, diced zucchini, and dried thyme. Sauté for 5 minutes.

Pour in chicken broth and bring to a boil. Simmer until vegetables are tender.

Season with salt and pepper, and serve this comforting turkey and vegetable soup.

Nutritional Benefits:

Turkey provides lean protein, and a variety of vegetables offer vitamins and minerals. This soup is hearty and satisfying for those with Crohn's disease.

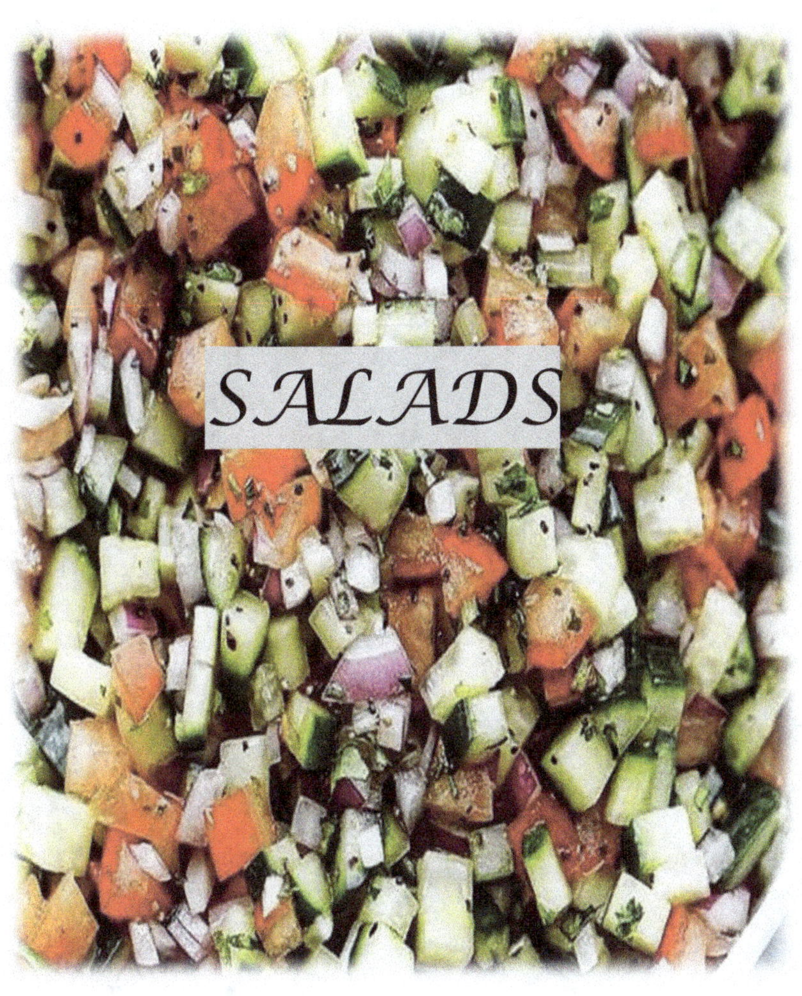

SALADS

Grilled Chicken and Quinoa Salad

Ingredients (for 2 servings):

1 cup cooked quinoa

2 boneless, skinless chicken breasts, grilled and sliced

2 cups mixed salad greens

1 cucumber, sliced

1 cup cherry tomatoes, halved

1/4 cup feta cheese, crumbled

Balsamic vinaigrette dressing

Salt and pepper to taste

Instructions:

In a large bowl, combine cooked quinoa, grilled chicken slices, salad greens, cucumber, and cherry tomatoes.

Toss the salad with balsamic vinaigrette dressing.

Sprinkle crumbled feta cheese on top.

Season with salt and pepper to taste.

Serve as a satisfying and protein-packed salad.

Nutritional Benefits:

Quinoa adds protein and fiber, while grilled chicken provides lean protein. Vegetables offer vitamins, and feta cheese adds a touch of creaminess.

Spinach and Strawberry Salad with Almonds

Ingredients (for 2 servings):

4 cups fresh spinach leaves

1 cup strawberries, sliced

1/4 cup almonds, sliced and toasted

1/2 avocado, diced

Feta cheese crumbles (optional)

Balsamic vinaigrette dressing

Salt and pepper to taste

Instructions:

In a large bowl, combine fresh spinach, sliced strawberries, toasted almonds, and diced avocado.

Toss the salad with balsamic vinaigrette dressing.

Add feta cheese crumbles if desired.

Season with salt and pepper to taste.

Enjoy this refreshing and nutrient-rich salad.

Nutritional Benefits:

Spinach provides vitamins and minerals, strawberries add antioxidants, and almonds contribute healthy fats and crunch.

Chickpea and Mediterranean Salad

Ingredients (for 2 servings):

1 can chickpeas, drained and rinsed

1 cucumber, diced

1 cup cherry tomatoes, halved

1/2 red onion, finely chopped

1/4 cup Kalamata olives, sliced

Feta cheese crumbles

Greek dressing

Fresh oregano for garnish

Salt and pepper to taste

Instructions:

In a bowl, combine chickpeas, diced cucumber, cherry tomatoes, chopped red onion, and sliced Kalamata olives.

Toss the salad with Greek dressing.

Sprinkle feta cheese crumbles on top.

Garnish with fresh oregano.

Season with salt and pepper to taste.

Serve as a flavorful and protein-rich Mediterranean salad.

Nutritional Benefits:

Chickpeas offer plant-based protein and fiber, while the Mediterranean flavors add a burst of taste. Olives provide healthy fats.

Salmon and Avocado Quinoa Salad

Ingredients (for 2 servings):

1 cup cooked quinoa

2 salmon fillets, grilled or baked

1 avocado, diced

1 cup cherry tomatoes, halved

2 cups mixed salad greens

Lemon vinaigrette dressing

Fresh dill for garnish

Salt and pepper to taste

Instructions:

In a large bowl, combine cooked quinoa, grilled salmon, diced avocado, cherry tomatoes, and mixed salad greens.

Toss the salad with lemon vinaigrette dressing.

Garnish with fresh dill.

Season with salt and pepper to taste.

Enjoy this omega-3 rich and satisfying salad.

Nutritional Benefits:

Quinoa provides protein and fiber, while salmon offers omega-3 fatty acids. Avocado adds healthy fats, and the salad greens offer vitamins.

Turkey and Cranberry Spinach Salad

Ingredients (for 2 servings):

2 cups fresh spinach leaves

1/2-pound turkey breast, sliced

1/4 cup dried cranberries

1/4 cup pecans, chopped and toasted

1/4 cup goat cheese, crumbled

Balsamic vinaigrette dressing

Salt and pepper to taste

Instructions:

In a large bowl, combine fresh spinach, sliced turkey breast, dried cranberries, and toasted pecans.

Toss the salad with balsamic vinaigrette dressing.

Sprinkle crumbled goat cheese on top.

Season with salt and pepper to taste.

Serve as a flavorful and protein-packed salad.

Nutritional Benefits:

Spinach provides vitamins and minerals, turkey adds lean protein, and cranberries contribute antioxidants. Pecans offer healthy fats.

Caprese Salad with Balsamic Glaze

Ingredients (for 2 servings):

2 large tomatoes, sliced

1 ball fresh mozzarella, sliced

Fresh basil leaves

Balsamic glaze

Extra virgin olive oil

Salt and pepper to taste

Instructions:

Arrange tomato and mozzarella slices alternately on a serving platter.

Tuck fresh basil leaves between the slices.

Drizzle with balsamic glaze and extra virgin olive oil.

Season with salt and pepper to taste.

Serve as a classic and refreshing Caprese salad.

Tomatoes provide lycopene, mozzarella offers calcium, and basil adds a burst of flavor. This salad is light and easy on the stomach.

Asian-Inspired Shrimp Salad

Ingredients (for 2 servings):

1/2-pound shrimp, peeled and deveined

2 cups shredded Napa cabbage

1 cup shredded carrots

1 bell pepper, thinly sliced

1/4 cup edamame, cooked

Sesame ginger dressing

Sesame seeds for garnish

Fresh cilantro for garnish

Salt and pepper to taste

Instructions:

In a pan, sauté shrimp until opaque and cooked through.

In a large bowl, combine shredded Napa cabbage, shredded carrots, sliced bell pepper, and cooked edamame.

Add the cooked shrimp to the salad.

Toss the salad with sesame ginger dressing.

Garnish with sesame seeds and fresh cilantro.

Season with salt and pepper to taste.

Serve as a light and flavorful Asian-inspired salad.

Nutritional Benefits:

Shrimp provides protein and omega-3 fatty acids. Napa cabbage and carrots add vitamins, and edamame contributes plant-based protein.

Mango and Chicken Quinoa Salad

Ingredients (for 2 servings):

1 cup cooked quinoa

1/2-pound chicken breast, grilled and sliced

1 mango, diced

1/2 cucumber, diced

1/4 cup red onion, finely chopped

Lime vinaigrette dressing

Fresh mint for garnish

Salt and pepper to taste

Instructions:

In a large bowl, combine cooked quinoa, grilled chicken slices, diced mango, diced cucumber, and finely chopped red onion.

Toss the salad with lime vinaigrette dressing.

Garnish with fresh mint.

Season with salt and pepper to taste.

Enjoy this tropical and protein-rich salad.

Nutritional Benefits:

Quinoa provides protein and fiber, while grilled chicken offers lean protein. Mango adds natural sweetness, and the salad is packed with vitamins.

Roasted Vegetable and Goat Cheese Salad

Ingredients (for 2 servings):

2 cups mixed salad greens

1 zucchini, sliced

1 red bell pepper, sliced

1/2 cup cherry tomatoes, halved

1/4 cup goat cheese, crumbled

Balsamic vinaigrette dressing

Fresh thyme for garnish

Salt and pepper to taste

Instructions:

Preheat the oven to 400°F (200°C).

Toss zucchini, red bell pepper, and cherry tomatoes with olive oil, salt, and pepper.

Roast the vegetables in the oven for 20-25 minutes or until tender.

In a bowl, combine mixed salad greens, roasted vegetables, and crumbled goat cheese.

Toss the salad with balsamic vinaigrette dressing.

Garnish with fresh thyme.

Serve as a flavorful and roasted vegetable-packed salad.

Nutritional Benefits:

Mixed salad greens provide vitamins, and roasted vegetables add a depth of flavor. Goat cheese contributes creaminess.

Egg Salad with Avocado and Greens

Ingredients (for 2 servings):

4 hard-boiled eggs, chopped

2 cups mixed salad greens

1 avocado, diced

1/4 cup radishes, sliced

2 tablespoons Greek yogurt

Dijon mustard to taste

Salt and pepper to taste

Fresh chives for garnish

Instructions:

In a bowl, combine chopped hard-boiled eggs, mixed salad greens, diced avocado, and sliced radishes.

In a separate bowl, mix Greek yogurt and Dijon mustard to create the dressing.

Toss the salad with the yogurt-Dijon dressing.

Season with salt and pepper to taste.

Garnish with fresh chives.

Serve as a protein-rich and creamy egg salad.

Nutritional Benefits:

Eggs provide protein, and avocado adds healthy fats. The Greek yogurt dressing is a lighter alternative to mayonnaise. Mixed greens offer vitamins and minerals.

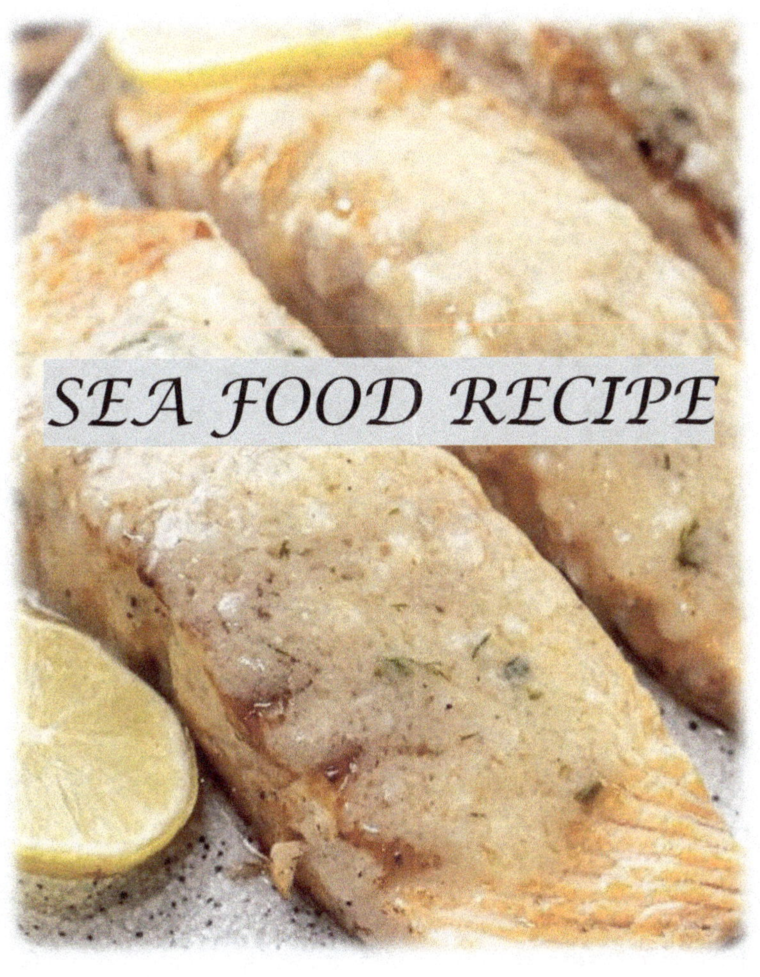

SEA FOOD RECIPE

Baked Lemon Garlic Salmon

Ingredients (for 2 servings):

2 salmon fillets

2 tablespoons olive oil

2 cloves garlic, minced

1 lemon, juiced

1 teaspoon dried oregano

Salt and pepper to taste

Fresh parsley for garnish

Instructions:

Preheat the oven to 400°F (200°C).

Place salmon fillets on a baking sheet.

In a small bowl, mix olive oil, minced garlic, lemon juice, dried oregano, salt, and pepper.

Brush the mixture over the salmon fillets.

Bake for 15-20 minutes or until the salmon flakes easily.

Garnish with fresh parsley before serving.

Nutritional Benefits:

Salmon provides omega-3 fatty acids, while garlic adds flavor without causing digestive distress.

Shrimp and Zucchini Noodles Stir-Fry

Ingredients (for 2 servings):

1/2-pound shrimp, peeled and deveined

2 zucchinis, spiralized into noodles

1 bell pepper, thinly sliced

2 tablespoons soy sauce (low sodium)

1 tablespoon sesame oil

1 tablespoon ginger, grated

2 cloves garlic, minced

Green onions for garnish

Sesame seeds for garnish

Instructions:

In a wok or large pan, heat sesame oil over medium-high heat.

Add shrimp, spiralized zucchini, and sliced bell pepper.

Stir-fry for 3-5 minutes or until shrimp is cooked.

Add soy sauce, grated ginger, and minced garlic. Stir well.

Garnish with green onions and sesame seeds before serving.

Nutritional Benefits:

Shrimp provides lean protein, and zucchini noodles offer a light and digestible alternative to traditional noodles.

Grilled Lemon Herb Tilapia

Ingredients (for 2 servings):

2 tilapia fillets

2 tablespoons olive oil

1 lemon, juiced

1 teaspoon dried thyme

1 teaspoon dried rosemary

Salt and pepper to taste

Fresh dill for garnish

Instructions:

Preheat the grill or grill pan.

Brush tilapia fillets with olive oil.

In a small bowl, mix lemon juice, dried thyme, dried rosemary, salt, and pepper.

Brush the lemon herb mixture over the tilapia fillets.

Grill for 3-4 minutes per side or until the fish is cooked through.

Garnish with fresh dill before serving.

Nutritional Benefits:

Tilapia is a mild fish that is easy to digest, and the lemon herb flavor adds a delicious touch.

Lemon Dijon Baked Cod

Ingredients (for 2 servings):

2 cod fillets

2 tablespoons Dijon mustard

1 lemon, juiced

1 tablespoon olive oil

1 teaspoon dried thyme

Salt and pepper to taste

Fresh parsley for garnish

Instructions:

Preheat the oven to 375°F (190°C).

Place cod fillets on a baking sheet.

In a small bowl, mix Dijon mustard, lemon juice, olive oil, dried thyme, salt, and pepper.

Spread the mixture over the cod fillets.

Bake for 15-20 minutes or until the fish is opaque and flakes easily.

Garnish with fresh parsley before serving.

Nutritional Benefits:

Cod is a mild fish that is well-tolerated, and the lemon Dijon flavor adds a zesty twist.

Tuna and Avocado Salad

Ingredients (for 2 servings):

1 can tuna, drained

1 avocado, diced

1 celery stalk, finely chopped

1/4 red onion, finely chopped

2 tablespoons Greek yogurt

1 tablespoon Dijon mustard

Salt and pepper to taste

Fresh dill for garnish

Instructions:

In a bowl, combine drained tuna, diced avocado, chopped celery, and chopped red onion.

In a small bowl, mix Greek yogurt, Dijon mustard, salt, and pepper.

Add the yogurt mixture to the tuna and toss until well combined.

Garnish with fresh dill before serving.

Serve as a light and protein-packed tuna salad.

Nutritional Benefits:

Tuna provides protein and omega-3 fatty acids, while avocado adds healthy fats and creaminess.

Sesame Ginger Scallops with Broccoli

Ingredients (for 2 servings):

1/2-pound scallops

1 cup broccoli florets

2 tablespoons soy sauce (low sodium)

1 tablespoon sesame oil

1 tablespoon ginger, grated

2 cloves garlic, minced

1 tablespoon sesame seeds for garnish

Green onions for garnish

Instructions:

In a wok or large pan, heat sesame oil over medium-high heat.

Add scallops and cook for 2-3 minutes on each side until golden brown.

Add broccoli florets, grated ginger, and minced garlic. Stir-fry for an additional 2-3 minutes.

Pour in soy sauce and toss until everything is well coated.

Garnish with sesame seeds and green onions before serving.

Nutritional Benefits:

Scallops provide protein, and broccoli adds fiber and essential nutrients. The sesame ginger flavor enhances the dish.

Lemon Butter Garlic Shrimp

Ingredients (for 2 servings):

1/2-pound shrimp, peeled and deveined

2 tablespoons unsalted butter

2 cloves garlic, minced

1 lemon, juiced

Fresh parsley for garnish

Salt and pepper to taste

Instructions:

In a skillet, melt butter over medium heat.

Add minced garlic and cook until fragrant.

Add shrimp to the skillet and cook for 2-3 minutes on each side until opaque.

Squeeze lemon juice over the shrimp.

Garnish with fresh parsley and season with salt and pepper before serving.

Shrimp provides lean protein, and the lemon butter garlic sauce adds richness without causing digestive distress.

Miso Glazed Salmon

Ingredients (for 2 servings):

2 salmon fillets

2 tablespoons white miso paste

1 tablespoon soy sauce (low sodium)

1 tablespoon mirin (sweet rice wine)

1 tablespoon honey

Sesame seeds for garnish

Green onions for garnish

Instructions:

Preheat the oven to 400°F (200°C).

In a small bowl, mix white miso paste, soy sauce, mirin, and honey to create the glaze.

Place salmon fillets on a baking sheet and brush the glaze over them.

Bake for 15-20 minutes or until the salmon is cooked through.

Garnish with sesame seeds and green onions before serving.

Nutritional Benefits:

Salmon provides omega-3 fatty acids, and the miso glaze adds a savory and umami flavor.

Cajun Spiced Snapper with Avocado Salsa

Ingredients (for 2 servings):

2 snapper fillets

1 tablespoon Cajun seasoning

1 tablespoon olive oil

1 avocado, diced

1 tomato, diced

1/4 red onion, finely chopped

Fresh cilantro for garnish

Lime wedges for serving

Salt and pepper to taste

Instructions:

Rub Cajun seasoning on both sides of snapper fillets.

In a skillet, heat olive oil over medium-high heat.

Cook snapper for 3-4 minutes on each side until the fish is opaque.

In a bowl, combine diced avocado, diced tomato, and finely chopped red onion to create the salsa.

Season the salsa with salt and pepper.

Serve snapper fillets topped with avocado salsa.

Garnish with fresh cilantro and serve with lime wedges.

Nutritional Benefits:

Snapper is a lean fish, and the Cajun spices add a flavorful kick. Avocado salsa provides healthy fats and freshness.

Lemon Herb Grilled Swordfish

Ingredients (for 2 servings):

2 swordfish steaks

2 tablespoons olive oil

1 lemon, juiced

1 teaspoon dried thyme

1 teaspoon dried rosemary

Salt and pepper to taste

Fresh chives for garnish

Instructions:

Preheat the grill or grill pan.

Brush swordfish steaks with olive oil.

In a small bowl, mix lemon juice, dried thyme, dried rosemary, salt, and pepper.

Brush the lemon herb mixture over the swordfish steaks.

Grill for 4-5 minutes per side or until the fish is cooked through.

Garnish with fresh chives before serving.

Nutritional Benefits:

Swordfish is a firm and meaty fish, and the lemon herb marinade adds a burst of flavor without overwhelming the digestive system.

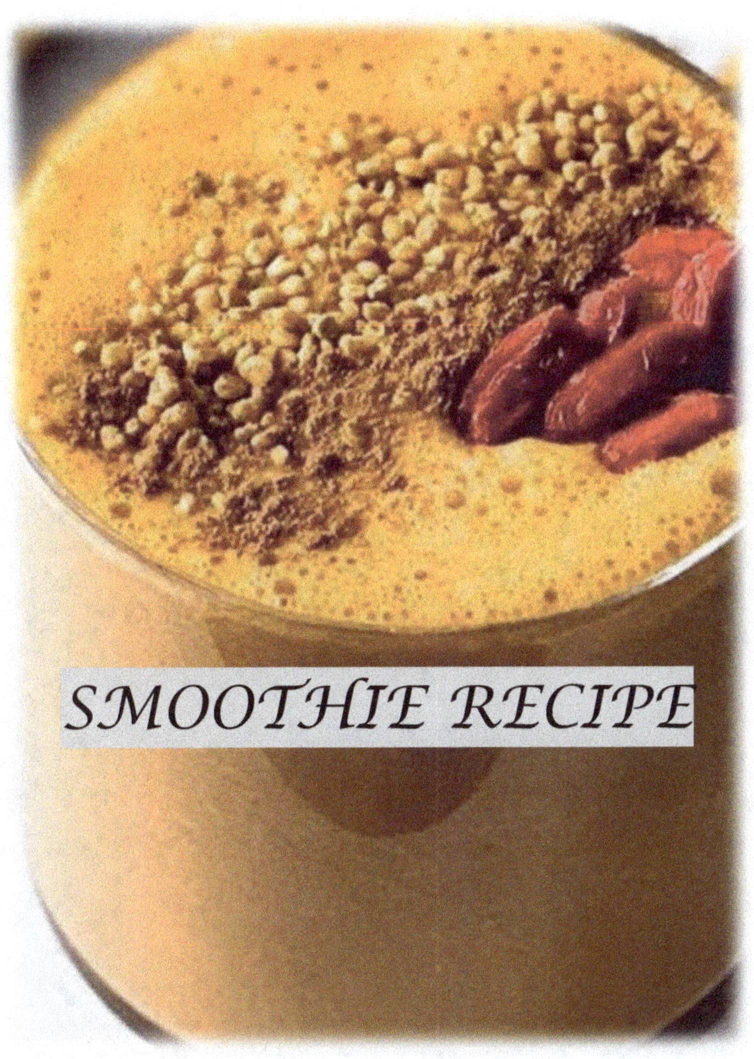

SMOOTHIE RECIPE

SMOOTHIES RECIPE

Banana Berry Bliss Smoothie

Ingredients (for 2 servings):

2 ripe bananas

1 cup mixed berries (strawberries, blueberries, raspberries)

1/2 cup Greek yogurt

1 cup almond milk (unsweetened)

1 tablespoon chia seeds

Ice cubes (optional)

Instructions:

Place bananas, mixed berries, Greek yogurt, almond milk, and chia seeds in a blender.

Blend until smooth and creamy.

Add ice cubes if a colder consistency is desired.

Pour into glasses and enjoy this antioxidant-rich smoothie.

Bananas offer potassium, berries provide antioxidants, Greek yogurt adds protein, and chia seeds contribute omega-3 fatty acids and fiber.

Mango Ginger Delight Smoothie

Ingredients (for 2 servings):

1 cup fresh or frozen mango chunks

1/2 cup plain kefir

1/2-inch fresh ginger, peeled and grated

1 tablespoon honey (optional)

1 cup coconut water

Handful of spinach (optional)

Ice cubes (optional)

Instructions:

Combine mango chunks, kefir, grated ginger, honey, coconut water, and spinach in a blender.

Blend until smooth and creamy.

Add ice cubes if desired for a refreshing texture.

Pour into glasses and savor the tropical goodness.

Nutritional Benefits:

Mangoes provide vitamins and natural sweetness, ginger aids digestion, kefir offers probiotics, and coconut water hydrates.

Green Goddess Detox Smoothie

Ingredients (for 2 servings):

1 cup kale leaves, stems removed

1/2 cucumber, peeled and sliced

1 green apple, cored and chopped

1/2 lemon, juiced

1 tablespoon flaxseeds

1 cup water or coconut water

Ice cubes (optional)

Instructions:

Combine kale leaves, cucumber, green apple, lemon juice, flaxseeds, and water in a blender.

Blend until smooth and detoxifying.

Add ice cubes if a colder temperature is preferred.

Pour into glasses and enjoy this nutrient-packed green smoothie.

Kale is rich in vitamins, cucumber hydrates, green apple adds natural sweetness, and flaxseeds offer omega-3 fatty acids and fiber.

Pineapple Mint Refresher Smoothie

Ingredients (for 2 servings):

1 cup fresh or frozen pineapple chunks

1/2 cup coconut milk (unsweetened)

Fresh mint leaves (to taste)

1 tablespoon honey (optional)

1/2 lime, juiced

1/2 teaspoon turmeric powder

Ice cubes (optional)

Instructions:

Blend pineapple chunks, coconut milk, fresh mint leaves, honey, lime juice, and turmeric powder until smooth.

Add ice cubes if a cooler consistency is desired.

Pour into glasses and enjoy this tropical and refreshing smoothie.

Nutritional Benefits:

Pineapple provides digestive enzymes, mint adds a burst of freshness, coconut milk offers healthy fats, and turmeric has anti-inflammatory properties.

Blueberry Almond Protein Smoothie

Ingredients (for 2 servings):

1 cup blueberries (fresh or frozen)

1/2 cup almond butter

1 cup almond milk (unsweetened)

1 scoop protein powder (unflavored or vanilla)

1 tablespoon chia seeds

Ice cubes (optional)

Instructions:

Blend blueberries, almond butter, almond milk, protein powder, and chia seeds until smooth.

Add ice cubes if a colder texture is preferred.

Pour into glasses and relish this protein-packed and satisfying smoothie.

Blueberries offer antioxidants, almond butter provides healthy fats, almond milk is lactose-free, and chia seeds contribute omega-3 fatty acids and fiber.

Carrot Cake Smoothie

Ingredients (for 2 servings):

1 cup carrots, peeled and chopped

1 banana

1/2 cup rolled oats

1/2 teaspoon cinnamon

1 cup almond milk (unsweetened)

1 tablespoon maple syrup or honey

Ice cubes (optional)

Instructions:

Blend chopped carrots, banana, rolled oats, cinnamon, almond milk, and maple syrup until smooth.

Add ice cubes if desired for a cooler sensation.

Pour into glasses and savor the flavors reminiscent of carrot cake.

Carrots provide beta-carotene, banana adds natural sweetness, rolled oats offer fiber, and cinnamon adds a warm and comforting touch.

Avocado Kale Power Smoothie

Ingredients (for 2 servings):

1/2 avocado, peeled and pitted

2 cups kale leaves, stems removed

1 cup pineapple chunks (fresh or frozen)

1 tablespoon chia seeds

1 cup coconut water

Ice cubes (optional)

Instructions:

Blend avocado, kale leaves, pineapple chunks, chia seeds, and coconut water until creamy.

Add ice cubes if a colder consistency is preferred.

Pour into glasses and enjoy this nutrient-dense and hydrating smoothie.

Nutritional Benefits:

Avocado offers healthy fats, kale is rich in vitamins, pineapple adds natural sweetness, and chia seeds contribute omega-3 fatty acids and fiber.

Strawberry Basil Citrus Smoothie

Ingredients (for 2 servings):

1 cup strawberries, hulled

1/2 cup fresh basil leaves

1 orange, peeled and segmented

1/2 lime, juiced

1 tablespoon honey (optional)

1 cup water or coconut water

Ice cubes (optional)

Instructions:

Blend strawberries, basil leaves, orange segments, lime juice, honey, and water until smooth.

Add ice cubes if a colder texture is desired.

Pour into glasses and relish this fruity and herb-infused smoothie.

Strawberries offer antioxidants, basil adds a unique flavor, citrus fruits provide vitamin C, and honey adds natural sweetness.

Raspberry Almond Chia Smoothie

Ingredients (for 2 servings):

1 cup raspberries (fresh or frozen)

1/2 cup almond milk (unsweetened)

2 tablespoons almond butter

1 tablespoon chia seeds

1 tablespoon honey (optional)

Ice cubes (optional)

Instructions:

Blend raspberries, almond milk, almond butter, chia seeds, and honey until smooth.

Add ice cubes if a colder consistency is preferred.

Pour into glasses and enjoy this delightful and nutty smoothie.

Nutritional Benefits:

Raspberries offer antioxidants, almond milk provides a dairy-free base, almond butter adds healthy fats, and chia seeds contribute omega-3 fatty acids and fiber.

Turmeric Mango Lassi Smoothie

Ingredients (for 2 servings):

1 cup mango chunks (fresh or frozen)

1 cup plain kefir or yogurt

1/2 teaspoon turmeric powder

1 tablespoon honey

1/2 teaspoon vanilla extract

Ice cubes (optional)

Instructions:

Blend mango chunks, kefir or yogurt, turmeric powder, honey, and vanilla extract until smooth.

Add ice cubes if a colder texture is desired.

Pour into glasses and savor the exotic and anti-inflammatory flavors.

Nutritional Benefits:

Mangoes provide vitamins and natural sweetness, kefir adds probiotics, turmeric has anti-inflammatory properties, and honey adds a touch of sweetness.

CHAPTER 3

TIPS ON MEAL PLANNING

Identify Trigger Foods:

Work with a healthcare professional to identify specific trigger foods that may exacerbate Crohn's symptoms. Common triggers include high-fiber foods, spicy foods, dairy, and certain raw fruits and vegetables.

Opt for Low-Fiber Options:

Choose easily digestible, low-fiber foods to reduce irritation to the digestive tract. Cook or steam vegetables to make them softer and more digestible.

Emphasize Lean Proteins:

Include lean proteins such as poultry, fish, eggs, and tofu. These are easier to digest and provide essential nutrients without causing excessive stress on the digestive system.

Incorporate Healthy Fats:

Include sources of healthy fats, such as avocados, olive oil, and nuts. These can provide essential nutrients and energy without irritating the digestive tract.

Consider Low-Lactose or Dairy-Free Options:

Many individuals with Crohn's disease have difficulty digesting lactose. Opt for lactose-free or dairy-free alternatives like almond milk, coconut milk, or lactose-free yogurt.

Limit Spices and Seasonings:

Minimize the use of spicy seasonings, as they can be harsh on the digestive system. Instead, use herbs like basil, mint, or dill for flavor without irritation.

Small, Frequent Meals:

Instead of large meals, consider smaller, more frequent meals throughout the day. This can help manage symptoms and prevent overloading the digestive system.

Hydration is Key:

Stay well-hydrated to support overall digestive health. Water is essential for maintaining hydration and aiding digestion.

Experiment with Food Preparation Techniques:

Experiment with cooking methods like baking, steaming, or boiling to make foods more easily digestible. These methods can help break down tough fibers in vegetables and meats.

Keep a Food Diary:

Track meals and symptoms in a food diary to identify patterns and connections between certain foods and symptom flare-ups. This can be valuable information for adjusting your diet.

Include Easily Digestible Carbohydrates:

Opt for easily digestible carbohydrates such as white rice, white potatoes, and refined grains. These are gentler on the digestive system.

Individualized Approach:

Crohn's disease can vary greatly between individuals. What works for one person may not work for another. Consider an individualized approach to meal planning based on personal tolerances and preferences.

Nutrient Supplementation:

Consult with a healthcare professional about potential nutrient deficiencies and whether supplementation is necessary. Crohn's disease can impact nutrient absorption.

Balance and Variety:

Strive for a balanced and varied diet to ensure a broad spectrum of nutrients. Rotate foods to prevent monotony and enhance nutritional intake.

Consult a Registered Dietitian:

Work closely with a registered dietitian who specializes in gastrointestinal disorders. They can provide personalized guidance, meal plans, and ongoing support.

TIPS ON GROCERY SHOPPING

Prepare a Shopping List:

Plan your meals in advance and create a detailed shopping list. This helps you stay focused on purchasing items that align with your dietary needs.

Shop the Perimeter:

The perimeter of the grocery store often contains fresh produce, lean proteins, and dairy alternatives. Stick to this area to find the majority of Crohn's-friendly ingredients.

Choose Fresh and Whole Foods:

Opt for fresh fruits, vegetables, lean meats, and whole grains. These foods are generally less processed and easier to digest.

Select Low-Fiber Options:

Choose low-fiber options for fruits and vegetables, such as peeled and cooked varieties. Canned or frozen fruits and vegetables can also be good alternatives.

Explore Gluten-Free Alternatives:

Consider gluten-free options for grains, such as rice, quinoa, and gluten-free oats. These can be gentler on the digestive system.

Dairy-Free and Lactose-Free Products:

Look for dairy-free or lactose-free alternatives, such as almond milk, coconut milk, or lactose-free yogurt.

Read Labels Carefully:

Check product labels for additives, preservatives, and high levels of sugar or artificial ingredients. Avoid items that may trigger symptoms.

Include Healthy Fats:

Choose sources of healthy fats like avocados, olive oil, and nuts. These provide essential nutrients without causing digestive distress.

Stock Up on Protein Sources:

Include lean protein sources such as poultry, fish, eggs, tofu, and plant-based proteins. Ensure that they are free from added marinades or spices that may be problematic.

Limit Processed Foods:

Minimize the purchase of heavily processed and packaged foods, as they may contain additives and preservatives that can be harsh on the digestive system.

Include Low-FODMAP Options:

For some individuals with Crohn's disease, following a low-FODMAP diet may be beneficial. Consider incorporating low-FODMAP options like certain fruits, vegetables, and grains.

Consider Nutrient Supplements:

If needed, include nutritional supplements recommended by a healthcare professional to address potential nutrient deficiencies.

Stock Up on Hydration:

Ensure you have an adequate supply of water or other hydrating beverages. Staying well-hydrated is crucial for digestive health.

Explore Alternative Grains:

Experiment with alternative grains like buckwheat, millet, and sorghum. These can provide variety in your diet.

Check for Allergens:

If you have additional food sensitivities or allergies, carefully check labels to avoid any potential triggers.

Plan for Small, Frequent Meals:

Purchase items suitable for creating smaller, more frequent meals throughout the day. This helps manage symptoms and prevents overloading the digestive system.

Frozen Fruits and Vegetables:

Consider purchasing frozen fruits and vegetables, as they can be just as nutritious and may have a longer shelf life.

Include Low-Residue Options:

Choose low-residue options, which are foods that are easily digestible and leave minimal residue in the colon. This can help manage symptoms during flares.

Check for Sale Flyers:

Look for sale flyers to take advantage of discounts on Crohn's-friendly staples. Consider buying in bulk when feasible.

Consult with a Dietitian:

If you have specific dietary concerns, consult with a registered dietitian specializing in gastrointestinal disorders. They can offer personalized guidance on grocery shopping and meal planning.

CONCLUSION

In the final pages of the **"Crohn's Disease Cookbook"** we embark on a journey that extends far beyond the kitchen – a journey of nourishment, empowerment, and embracing a life well-lived despite the challenges of Crohn's disease. As we conclude this culinary exploration, it is essential to reflect on the significance of this cookbook in the lives of those touched by this chronic condition.

The pages preceding this conclusion have been filled with carefully curated recipes, thoughtful meal planning tips, and strategic grocery shopping guidance, all tailored to cater to the unique needs of individuals grappling with Crohn's disease. Through the lens of nutrition and mindful culinary choices, we have aimed not only to alleviate symptoms but to empower individuals to take an active role in managing their health.

As we bid farewell to these pages, it is our sincere hope that the **"Crohn's Disease Cookbook"** becomes more than just a kitchen companion – it evolves into a source of inspiration, a guide through the ups and downs of managing dietary challenges, and a reminder that delicious and healing can indeed coexist on a plate.

To our readers, we extend gratitude for entrusting us with a small part of your journey. May the recipes within these pages bring not only culinary delight but also a sense of empowerment, allowing you to reclaim control over your well-being. Remember, each meal prepared from this cookbook is a step towards a healthier, more vibrant life.

In closing, let the "Crohn's Disease Cookbook" be a reminder that, despite the intricacies of managing this condition, there is beauty and strength in the act of nourishing oneself. The kitchen, once a potential source of anxiety, is now a space for creativity, healing, and a celebration of the resilience that defines each individual on this journey.

Bon appétit to a life enriched with flavors, nurtured by understanding, and seasoned with the unwavering spirit of those who face Crohn's disease with courage and grace.

DAILY MEAL PLANNER

DAILY MEAL PLANNER

DAY/DATE: ______________________________

BREAKFAST

GROCERY LIST

LUNCH

DINNER

SNACKS

NOTES

DAILY MEAL PLANNER

DAY/DATE: ___________________________

BREAKFAST

GROCERY LIST

LUNCH

DINNER

SNACKS

NOTES

DAILY MEAL PLANNER

DAY/DATE: _______________________________

BREAKFAST

LUNCH

DINNER

SNACKS

GROCERY LIST

NOTES

DAILY MEAL PLANNER

DAY/DATE: _______________________

BREAKFAST

LUNCH

DINNER

GROCERY LIST

SNACKS

NOTES

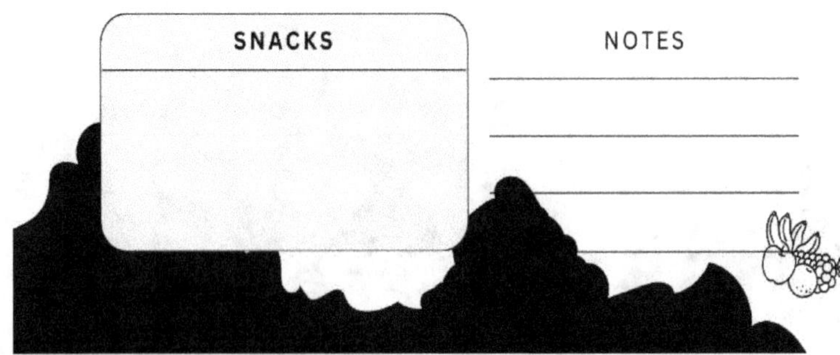

DAILY MEAL PLANNER

DAY/DATE: _______________________

BREAKFAST

GROCERY LIST

LUNCH

DINNER

SNACKS

NOTES

DAILY MEAL PLANNER

DAY/DATE: _______________________________

BREAKFAST

LUNCH

DINNER

GROCERY LIST

SNACKS

NOTES

DAILY MEAL PLANNER

DAY/DATE: ______________________________

BREAKFAST

GROCERY LIST

LUNCH

DINNER

SNACKS

NOTES

DAILY MEAL PLANNER

DAY/DATE: _______________________________

BREAKFAST

GROCERY LIST

LUNCH

DINNER

SNACKS

NOTES

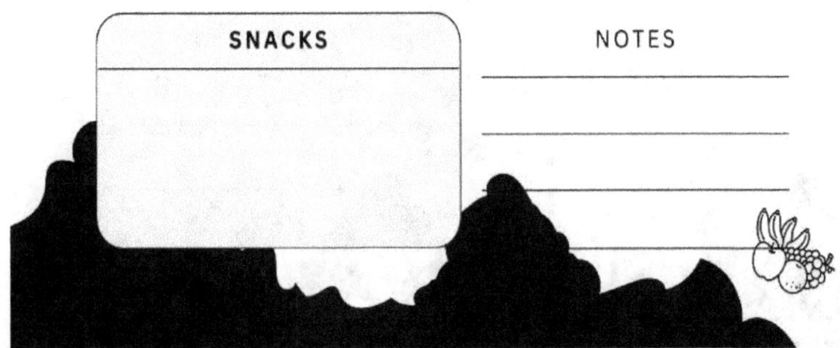

DAILY MEAL PLANNER

DAY/DATE: _______________________________

BREAKFAST

GROCERY LIST

LUNCH

DINNER

SNACKS

NOTES

DAILY MEAL PLANNER

DAY/DATE: _______________________________

BREAKFAST

GROCERY LIST

LUNCH

DINNER

SNACKS

NOTES

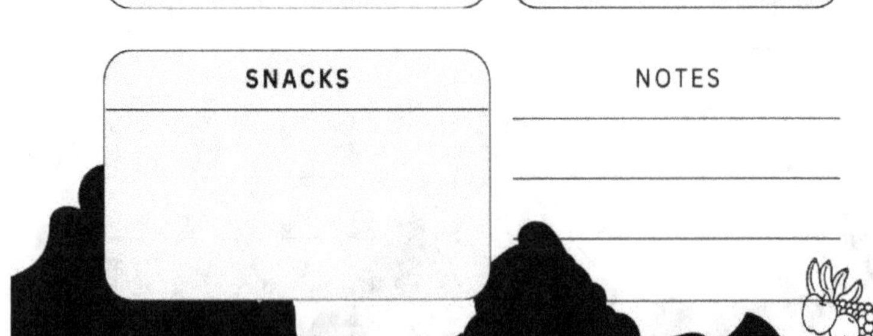

DAILY MEAL PLANNER

DAY/DATE: _______________________

BREAKFAST

LUNCH

DINNER

GROCERY LIST

SNACKS

NOTES

DAILY MEAL PLANNER

DAY/DATE: _______________________

BREAKFAST

GROCERY LIST

LUNCH

DINNER

SNACKS

NOTES

DAILY MEAL PLANNER

DAY/DATE: ______________________________

BREAKFAST

GROCERY LIST

LUNCH

DINNER

SNACKS

NOTES

DAILY MEAL PLANNER

DAY/DATE: _______________________

BREAKFAST

GROCERY LIST

LUNCH

DINNER

SNACKS

NOTES

DAILY MEAL PLANNER

DAY/DATE: _______________________

BREAKFAST

GROCERY LIST

LUNCH

DINNER

SNACKS

NOTES

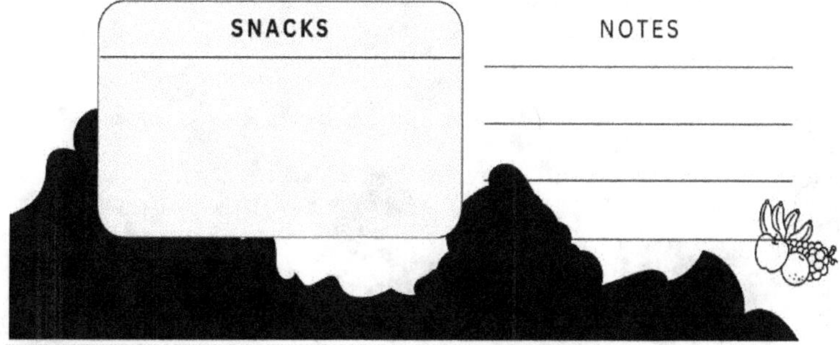

DAILY MEAL PLANNER

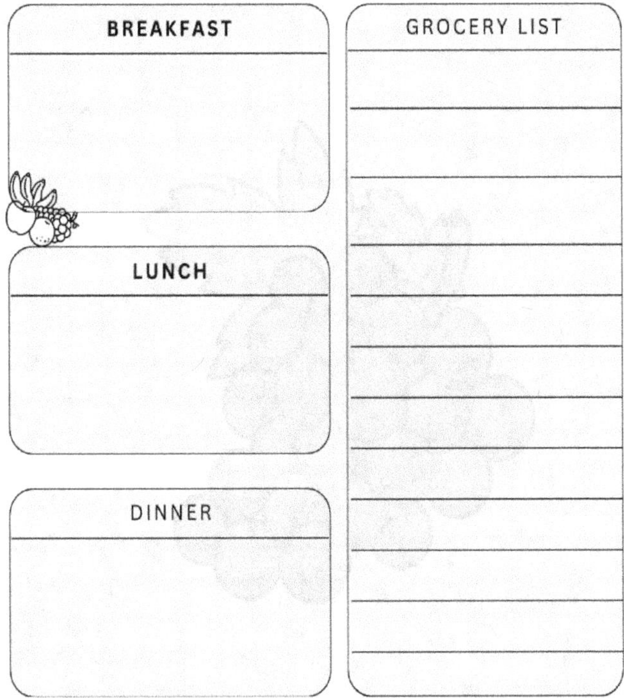

DAY/DATE: _______________________

BREAKFAST

LUNCH

DINNER

GROCERY LIST

SNACKS

NOTES

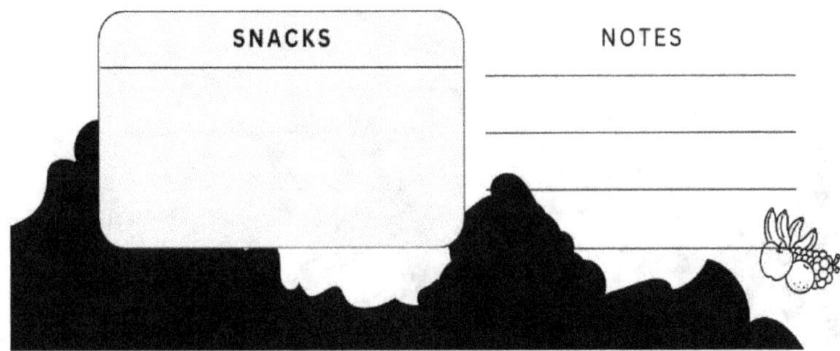

DAILY MEAL PLANNER

DAY/DATE: _______________________

BREAKFAST

GROCERY LIST

LUNCH

DINNER

SNACKS

NOTES

DAILY MEAL PLANNER

DAY/DATE: _______________________

BREAKFAST

GROCERY LIST

LUNCH

DINNER

SNACKS

NOTES
____
____
____

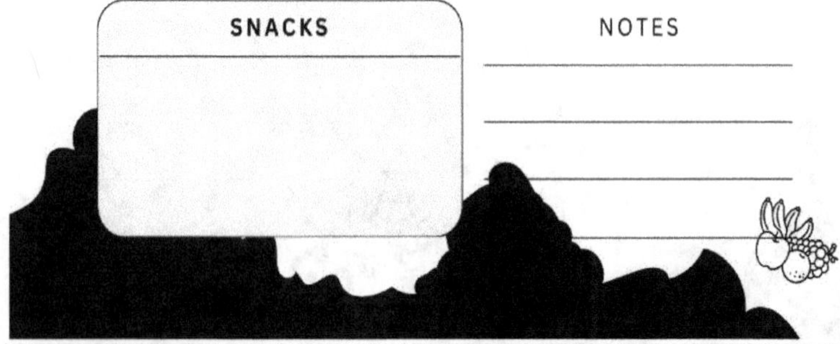

DAILY MEAL PLANNER

DAY/DATE: _______________________________

BREAKFAST

GROCERY LIST

LUNCH

DINNER

SNACKS

NOTES

DAILY MEAL PLANNER

DAY/DATE: _______________________________

BREAKFAST

GROCERY LIST

LUNCH

DINNER

SNACKS

NOTES

DAILY MEAL PLANNER

DAY/DATE: _______________________________

BREAKFAST

GROCERY LIST

LUNCH

DINNER

SNACKS

NOTES

DAILY MEAL PLANNER

DAY/DATE: _______________________________

BREAKFAST

LUNCH

DINNER

GROCERY LIST

SNACKS

NOTES

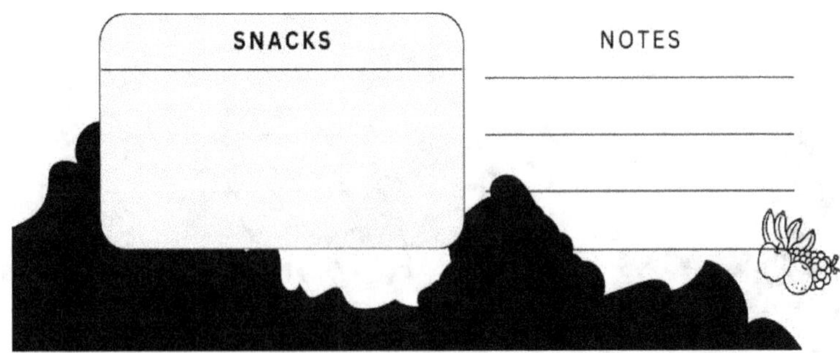

DAILY MEAL PLANNER

DAY/DATE: ___________________________

BREAKFAST

GROCERY LIST

LUNCH

DINNER

SNACKS

NOTES

DAILY MEAL PLANNER

DAY/DATE: ___________________________

BREAKFAST

GROCERY LIST

LUNCH

DINNER

SNACKS

NOTES

DAILY MEAL PLANNER

DAY/DATE: _______________________________

BREAKFAST

GROCERY LIST

LUNCH

DINNER

SNACKS

NOTES

DAILY MEAL PLANNER

DAY/DATE: _______________________

BREAKFAST

GROCERY LIST

LUNCH

DINNER

SNACKS

NOTES

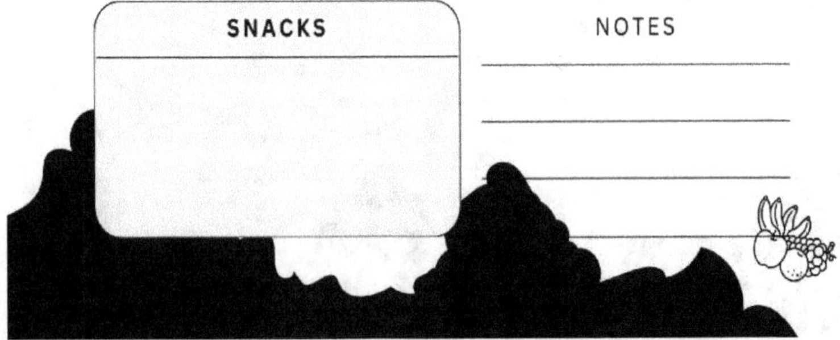

DAILY MEAL PLANNER

DAY/DATE: ___________________________

BREAKFAST

GROCERY LIST

LUNCH

DINNER

SNACKS

NOTES

DAILY MEAL PLANNER

DAY/DATE: _______________________________

BREAKFAST

LUNCH

DINNER

GROCERY LIST

SNACKS

NOTES

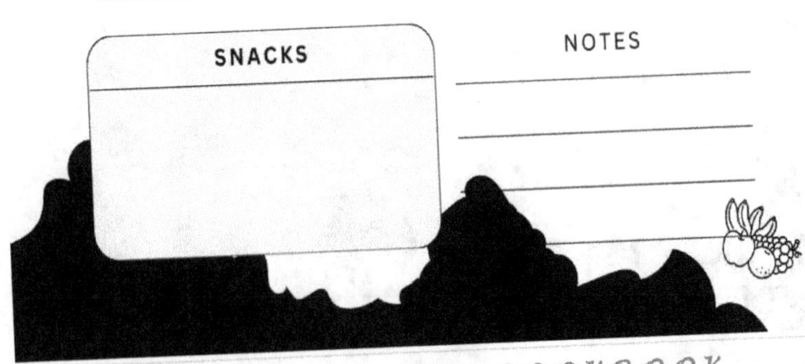

DAILY MEAL PLANNER

DAY/DATE: ___________________________

BREAKFAST

GROCERY LIST

LUNCH

DINNER

SNACKS

NOTES

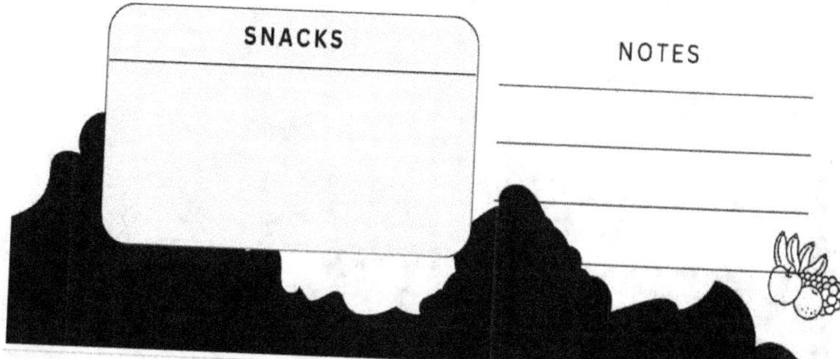

DAILY MEAL PLANNER

DAY/DATE: _______________________

BREAKFAST

GROCERY LIST

LUNCH

DINNER

SNACKS

NOTES

www.ingramcontent.com/pod-product-compliance
Lightning Source LLC
Chambersburg PA
CBHW070828250726
48662CB00003B/1124